DIMENSIONS OF THE HEALING MINISTRY

JAMES E. HUG, SJ
Editor

In association with the Center of Concern

The Catholic Health Association of the United States
St. Louis, MO

Copyright © 1989
by
The Catholic Health Association of the United States
4455 Woodson Road
St. Louis, MO 63134-0889

Library of Congress Cataloging-in-Publication Data

Hug, James E.
    Dimensions of the healing ministry/James E. Hug in association with the Center of Concern.
        p.   cm.
    Includes bibliographies and index.
    ISBN 0-87125-170-1
    1. Church work with the sick. 2. Pastoral medicine—Catholic Church. 3. Medicine—Religious aspects—Catholic Church. 4. Health—Religious aspects—Catholic Church. 5. Catholic Church–United States—Charities. 6. Catholic Church—Doctrines.
        I. Center of Concern (Washington, D.C.) II. Title.
        [DNLM: 1. Catholicism. 2. Pastoral Care. 3. Religion and Medicine. W 50 H891d]
    BX2347.8.S5H84   1989
    261.8'321—dc19
    DNLM/DLC
    for Library of Congress   89-896
                                                                  CIP

Contents

Foreword

Are you ready to think about how Jesus Christ would have acted if, instead of sending his son to live in the Middle East two thousand years ago as a carpenter, God sent his son to live in the United States today as a doctor, nurse, hospital administrator, home health aide, bedpan cleaner, hospital chaplain, healthcare insurer, trustee of a hospital, organizer of a hospital union, or a poor or wealthy patient?

If you are, you'll have the time of your life reading this book and reflecting on the pointed questions it raises.

If you're not, or if you expect clear answers to the devilishly difficult choices that confront those who choose a role in the Catholic healthcare ministry, then go back to catechism by rote. For this is a series of essays for those who are serious enough about instilling moral values into the American healthcare system to think through practical ways to get the job done.

Above all, these essays beg us to remember that, among all the marvelous medicines and machines, amidst the modern hospital centers with their Buck Rogers operating rooms and Star Wars intensive care units, among all the unclear scanners and brutal chemotherapy, the radiation and tubes and gadgets that can mimic just about every organ—among all these mechanical and chemical miracles—access to healthcare, even at its most basic, is central to the human dignity that Christ has asked us to accord the least among us.

This book roams over a wide range of topics and probes the responsibilities of all sorts of healthcare providers. But a common theme drives its authors: You Christians who would devote all or part of your life and time to healthcare are not simply in the healthcare industry (important as efficient and business-like management are), you are in the healthcare ministry, whose work is distinguished and inspired by the recognition that helping the sick and the injured is giving them a better chance to live the way they were created to live, in the image of God.

Reflecting on the many penetrating and vexing questions this book raises, I was reminded of two incidents that taught me more about healthcare than the thousands of pages of material I studied during my years as Secretary of Health, Education, and Welfare, or my years since, wrestling with the slippery, sinewy cost monster that threatens the very viability of America's healthcare system.

On the early evening of November 10, 1978, I met at his residence with the heroic Polish prelate, Stefan Cardinal Wyszynski, a meeting the Polish government had unsuccessfully attempted to block. The Cardinal's presence was powerful enough to fill the room, despite the weakness of his quiet voice. "There are too many machines and tubes and wires," he said. "Even with the best machines, people often die or remain sick because they have no human contact, because they do not touch other people. People need contact to be cured."

The Cardinal paused for a moment, then continued, "A machine saved my life some time ago, but I am still concerned about the use of machines without adequate human contact. Even when one goes to the dentist, there are too many machines. When I was in Rome some time ago, there were so many cables and wires and electric machines that I asked the dentist if he needed those just to fix a tooth. The dentist replied that today, everyone had such machinery. But the machinery he was using could have killed us both."

The Cardinal asked me if the doctors I had met in Poland or knew in the United States were sensitive to "the need for one person to touch another." As I was leaving and we faced each other in his dimly lit foyer, he said, "You are the Minister of Health. When you go back home I hope you will urge doctors in the United States to recognize how important human contact is."

The other incident occurred on the air shuttle from New York to Washington in 1985. I was sitting in the same row with Vernon Jordan, the courageous civil rights leader with whom I had worked when he was registering Southern voters in the 1960s and I was one of President Lyndon Johnson's assistants. Jordan was now a Washington lawyer, and a few years before he had been seriously wounded by a shot in the back one evening as he entered a hotel. "You know what kept me alive, Joe," he said, "It wasn't the skill of the doctor—though he was superb. It was the fact that he held my hand for the better part of three days, there in the hospital, just holding my hand, that touching is why I survived."

On those Fridays when we're in Washington, my wife Hilary works as a volunteer at Georgetown Hospital's Lombardi Cancer Center. When I asked her what she does, she said simply, "I talk to the patients who are awaiting chemotherapy or who have just received it." When I asked her, "About what?" She said, "About whatever is on their mind." The head of the medical center at Georgetown told me that the women who do this are as important to those frightened patients and their health as any chemical, any machine, any doctor, or any fully trained nurse. It is, after all, another way of touching.

The authors of this volume insist that healthcare is indeed a ministry. Their book will disturb many readers with its suggestions that too often Catholic healthcare, caught up in the day-to-day problems of rising costs in a secular society, has acted like an industry; its demand that we at least ask the question whether we should continue to build and buy so many expensive machines when we have more than 35 million Americans without adequate healthcare; its questions about the relations between labor and management in the special context of the Catholic healthcare ministry; its spotlight on whether an individual with the wealth to maintain life at incredible cost (often a life of only marginal quality) has the moral right to spend so much money to live tied to tubes and machines, while children in ghettos and around the world go without basic care; its push to get Catholics in healthcare to let the big secret of Church teaching on social responsibility and the U.S. Bishops pastoral letter, *Health and Health Care,* out of the closet and into their lives.

For me the essays drive home the moral imperative of stemming healthcare inflation and profligate medical practices, of eliminating useless procedures, of finding out what works under what circumstances, of limiting intrusions into the human body—which, after all, houses our souls while we are on earth and is the vehicle through which we are to "know, love and serve God"—to circumstances where they are necessary to maintain or restore health. What we waste on unnecessary procedures, on neighboring hospitals keeping-up-with-the-Joneses by excessive exotic equipment purchases, on self-inflicted illness due to smoking, excessive drinking, and gluttony, adds up to more than enough money to provide healthcare for all our indigent citizens. Here the issue is not the way, but the will. We know how. Do we care to?

This volume is also a poignant reminder of the dignity of human labor, of the reality that doing a common thing uncommonly well brings success.

We have a nursing shortage in America. There is also a critical need for home health aides. The shortages of people to care for the elderly are serious enough to add fuel to the early flames of those who would resort to euthanasia to slow the costs of the aging of America. We are too quick to attribute these shortages to inadequate pay. Pay may well be a problem in a materialistic society. But I believe there is a far more profound reason for these shortages.

There is no need to pay a mother or a father to take care of their children. But when we ask adult children, or their surrogates, to provide the same care for the elderly—bathing, toileting, feeding, assisting to walk, companionship—the answer is increasingly, No. This is a question of values, yes, and also of the fact that we have not accorded to tasks such as nursing and home healthcare the dignity which they deserve.

That such work is the work of God every Christian knows well. That such work is Christ-like, we all learned from reading the Gospels and listening to a thousand Sunday sermons. That such work lays bricks on the road to heaven, every Catholic would attest.

It's time for more than lip service. We need to recognize by how we treat, what we pay, how we honor those who tend to our sick and elderly, those who do the messy jobs of human caring, that their work is just as dignified and important as any other of the healthcare vocations, or any of the so-called loftier tasks of manufacturing, investing, lawyering, teaching, governing. By the time you put this book down, you will understand, as never before, how pressing is that need.

Joseph A. Califano, Jr.
Washington, DC
Fall 1989

Introduction

Catholic healthcare is a highly significant expression of church ministry today. Millions of people and billions of dollars are committed to serving the sick and the dying, the elderly, and all who suffer in so many ways. In their 1981 pastoral letter, *Health and Health Care*, the U.S. bishops emphasized that this service continues Jesus' healing ministry:

> Members of the church follow the example of Jesus, therefore, when they carry out the work of healing— not only by providing care for the physically ill, but also by working to restore health and wholeness in all facets of the human person and the human community.[1]

The history of Catholic involvement in healthcare is a proud element of the church's ministerial tradition. It is a history of moving compassion and deeply committed competence, but it is also a history whose future contains serious questions.

Two very significant challenges have emerged in recent years. Concern over healthcare costs has generated severe economic pressures on healthcare institutions, resulting in a growing emphasis on an industrial model of management that gives extremely high priority to the value of economic efficiency. Second, there are fewer sponsoring religious communities, leading to a significant change in the key personnel who embody and shape the spirit of Catholic healthcare institutions.

The industrial model of healthcare management is becoming prominent nationwide, both in the "for-profit" and the "nonprofit" sectors. In an effort to become more competitive, many institutions now emphasize managerial approaches drawn from the industrial world that seem to endanger the traditional person-centered ministerial focus that has characterized Catholic healthcare for so long. Although the commitment to serving the poor still receives strong support among Catholic healthcare providers, it is slipping dangerously close to drowning in red ink. Increasingly we hear the slogan, "No margin, no mission." Others object that there is no reason to struggle so hard to scrape out a margin if we end up sacrificing our mission in the process. The mission is not what is achieved after expenses are met. This challenge is deathly serious.

It is also a challenge with far reaching implications for the Judeo-Christian tradition. Can people who adhere faithfully to Judeo-Christian values survive and thrive in the U.S. political economy? At a time when the U.S. bishops are calling us all to see our work as a vocation, as our response to God's personal call to each of us, those who have long defined their work in vocational and ministerial language are being submitted to the pressures of capitalism's marketplace as never before. Healthcare providers stand as heralds to the rest of our society of the feasibility of the struggle for fidelity to Christian social values in the contemporary capitalist world.

Another important challenge influencing the future of Catholic healthcare is the changing character of the personnel involved in key administrative, supervisory, and staff positions. Members of religious communities are no longer the dominant presence in Catholic institutions and systems. The age of the laity is emerging in healthcare as it is elsewhere throughout the church. The ministerial values that have long been the heart of Catholic healthcare must now be carried preeminently by the lay women and men who serve there.

The laity bring with them a spirituality capable of greatly enriching healthcare ministry today. But it is part of the tragic failure of adult religious formation in the Catholic church that too few have consciously developed their spirituality or learned to be confident in its capacities for guiding their personal and institutional activities.

It is important, then, that all who are connected with healthcare ministry—especially those in positions of leadership—continually develop themselves in the values and visions that characterized the founding of Catholic healthcare institutions, those responsive to the needs of the present, and those the future will demand. The spirit of ministry must be actively nurtured and developed constantly.

These two major challenges promise to transform the character of Catholic healthcare in the next decade. The outcome is far from clear. The days ahead will require a great deal of prayer, reflection, and courageous action. This book is intended to help in that process. It attempts to clarify the contemporary context within which these developments are occurring, to contribute to the formation of the kind of courageous, lifegiving faith identity healthcare providers need, to raise some of the hard questions that must be faced, to suggest processes for prayerful discernment, and to point in some of the new, alternative directions that we see as important. Its four main sections each have a brief introduction providing a hint of the chapters' themes. Each chapter is followed by questions for reflection and discussion.

The ideas here have been developed in dialogue with a variety of Catholic healthcare communities. We owe our gratitude to The Catholic Health Association, CHA Wisconsin, Mercy Health Services, the Sisters of Providence Corporation of Seattle, the Holy Cross Health System of South Bend, The Bon Secours Health System, The CHAP Program, Wheaton Franciscan Services, Inc., The National Association of Catholic Chaplains, and *Health Progress* for providing the opportunities and arenas for this ongoing discussion.

We deeply appreciate the fine Foreword prepared by Joseph Califano. It reflects a careful, insightful reading of the text and a passionate commitment to its values. We are sincerely grateful.

In addition, several organizations provided grants that helped make this volume possible. We want to thank publicly The Sisters of Mercy Health System, The Franciscan Sisters of the Poor Health System, Inc., The Catholic Medical Center of Brooklyn and Queens, Inc., The Sisters of Mercy Health System of St. Louis, The Franciscan Sisters of Honolulu, and The Sisters of Providence Corporate Headquarters.

I want to thank Sr. Normandie Gaitley, SSJ, for her help in preparing the reflection questions that follow each chapter and for her enthusiastic support for this project. Finally, Judy Mladineo dedicated endless hours to the seemingly infinite number of details required to turn these pages into a polished manuscript. She also prepared the fine index. She deserves deep and sincere gratitude from all of us—writers and readers alike.

James E. Hug, SJ
Center of Concern

1. *Health and Health Care,* National Conference of Catholic Bishops, *Origins,* Vol. 11, No. 25, Dec. 3, 1981, p. 397.

The Challenge Today

Religiously based, church-affiliated healthcare institutions have experienced notable changes in the past 20 years. To respond adequately to future challenges in the spirit of Jesus, Catholic healthcare leaders must be aware of the larger world that is daily shaping healthcare and that desperately needs healthcare's healing ministry. No activity—not even the most complex medical specialization—can be separated from the context within which it functions and in relationship with which it draws its meaning and value.

Chapter 1 delineates a few economic, political, ecclesial, technological, and social dimensions of today's world. It points out that if we respond to this world based on the Judeo-Christian tradition's social vision and values, we will need to pursue a new "path" in healthcare ministry—a path demanding some challenging personal, professional, and organizational commitments from us all.

· 1 ·

Building a Healthy Society:
A Catholic Challenge of the Future[1]

Peter J. Henriot, SJ

In a biblical understanding of stewardship, the good and faithful
steward is one who provides well for the future. In today's world—a
world in which "the future is not what it used to be"—we must all
be good and faithful stewards. This is especially true of those
blessed with the vocation of serving people through the healthcare ministry.

In this chapter, I want to make three major points. The
challenge for the future facing Catholic healthcare involves a
context, a *content,* and a *consequence.* In discussing the context, I will
sketch some dimensions currently unfolding in the world, the
church, and the healthcare field. In discussing the content, I will
outline those themes of our Catholic/Christian tradition that can
and should guide our movement into the future. And in discussing
the consequence, I will suggest the central direction that I feel is
necessary to shape the future.

Before addressing these topics, however, let me emphasize that I assume the following regarding people involved in
religiously based healthcare:

You are committed to healthcare ministry, not to healthcare *industry.* As heirs of a tradition established in this country
largely through the imaginative and courageous efforts of women
and men religious, you are "in the business" not "for the sake of
business" but to share in the healing mission of Jesus Christ and

his church, the Christian community. As the 1981 pastoral letter of the U.S. bishops, *Health and Health Care,* states quite clearly: "Members of the church follow the example of Jesus, therefore, when they carry out the work of healing—not only by providing care for the physically ill, but also by working to restore health and wholeness in all facets of the human person and human community."[2]

However much the language of industrial organization may enter into your discussion—corporations, systems analysis, chief executive officer, delivery systems, strategic planning, and consumers, the industrial model, with its accompanying values of cost-effectiveness, competition, and, growth, is not your primary model. Others may be engaged in healthcare industry; you, as members of religiously based healthcare institutions, are engaged in health-care ministry.

The Context

"The whole human race faces a moment of supreme crisis in its advance toward maturity."[3] With these words, quoted from the Second Vatican Council, the U.S. Roman Catholic bishops open their pastoral letter on war and peace. I was in Chicago when that Pastoral Letter, *The Challenge of Peace: God's Promise and Our Response,* was approved. I know the sense, the premonition, that what the bishops had accomplished—in process as well as in product—was going to have ripples, implications far beyond the issue of war and peace.

The healing ministry today moves into the future at "a moment of supreme crisis." Some of the future that I see unfolding before us can be described under the headings of world, church, and healthcare.

In the World

We are moving very precariously toward the year 2000. Indeed, we may not reach the year 2000 without major changes in our patterns and structures for doing things. We are faced, for example, with the twin threats of global poverty and the arms race.

We live on a globe where the World Bank estimates that nearly half the population—2.5 billion of 5 billion inhabitants—live in nations with an annual gross national product (GNP) per capita of less than $400.[4] In 1980, then World Bank President Robert McNamara reported that at least 800 million people in those countries live in situations of absolute poverty, "beneath any rational definition of human decency."[5] An estimated 44,000 people a day die of starvation and malnutrition. The U.S. Catholic bishops' pastoral on the economy comments:

> Nearly half a billion are chronically hungry, despite abundant harvests world-wide. Fifteen out of every 100 children born in those countries die before the age of five, and millions of the survivors are physically or mentally stunted. No aggregate of individual examples could portray adequately the appalling inequities within those desperately poor countries and between them and our own. And their misery is not the inevitable result of the march of history or of the intrinsic nature of particular cultures, but of human decisions and human institutions.[6]

The world's population is doubling now every 35 or 40 years, and 90 percent of that doubling goes on amidst the hungry and poor of Asia, Latin America, and Africa. Of the more than a billion people who will be added to the world's population before the year 2000, more than half will be in the poorest countries, those with a GNP of less than $400 per capita.[7] We refer to these nations as the "Third World," but they clearly constitute the "Two-Thirds World." Of course, there is no need to go abroad to see poverty of that magnitude since it is also present in the urban and rural areas of this country, in which we live and minister.

If worsening global poverty were not enough to sober us, there is the arms race and the consequent threat of nuclear war. We have all paid increasing attention to that fact in recent months and years. We have seen the expenditure of $900 billion a year worldwide for armaments[8] and a U.S. defense budget during the Reagan Administration of well over $1.5 trillion. We have seen that if a button were pushed in Moscow launching a Soviet ICBM targeted on your city, you would not have time to finish this chapter. We have seen the reality of six nations publicly holding nuclear arms today, the possibility that two or three other nations secretly hold them, and the probability that in 15 years 20 more nations will hold them, plus various terrorist groups. This twin threat hovers over our world today, the world wherein you exercise your healthcare ministry.

In the Church

We continue to face the great challenge of implementing the reform and renewal mandated by the Second Vatican Council. We have all experienced the profound changes instituted by the council—in liturgy, ecumenism, the role of the laity, moral teaching, education, ministry, and so on. We have experienced the turmoil and pain, as well as the progress and joy.

The Catholic church's process of self-identification has had two significant marks: (1) it is a *community*, with the images of the People of God, the pilgrim church; and (2) it is *engaged in the world*, not separate or isolated but involved in promoting justice and peace. Shaping that self-identification at this very moment is the phenomenal growth of church membership outside of the North Atlantic community (Europe and North America). As the German theologian Karl Rahner has emphasized, we see a truly "world church" taking shape wherein the vital theologies, liturgies, and communities of Africa, Latin America, and Asia will increasingly influence what we call Roman Catholicism.[9]

Another influential force shaping today's church is the present Pope's personality and style. Intellectual, charismatic, non-Italian, highly political, and widely traveled, Pope John Paul II has and will continue to have a great impact on the church's future.

Another highly influential factor in the church of the future will be the laity's role. Called to exercise greater responsibilities, the laity are assuming more important positions every day. This will certainly be true in healthcare ministry, where fewer and fewer women and men religious are available. Those who have watched the composition of The Catholic Health Association change over the last 20 years can imagine how it will look after 10 years. The consequences of current trends are very clear.

In the Field of Healthcare

This context is certainly changing rapidly as the future unfolds. I am aware from the work of the Center of Concern, a consultant to several Catholic healthcare organizations, that U.S. healthcare is feeling the impact of government decisions, economic conditions, technological breakthroughs, and changing values. As sociologist Paul Starr notes in his monumental work *The Social Transformation of American Medicine,* "Medicine, like many other American institutions, suffered a stunning confidence loss in the 1970s."[10] The public began seriously questioning the value of medical care and the desirability of allowing physicians and their allies to have the primary say in running healthcare systems.

A number of emerging issues will challenge healthcare ministry as we know it today. Clement Bezold, director of the Washington-based Institute for Alternative Futures, notes five of them:

1. *The increasing proportion of the elderly.* Current popula-tion trends indicate that the proportion of those over age 65 will rise significantly in the next few decades (from about 11 percent in the mid-1980s to nearly 18 percent by 2020). This will sharply increase the demand for hospital care for the elderly as well as spur development of noninstitutional approaches to care.
2. *The communications revolution.* Developments in tele-vision, telephones, and computers will mean that per-sonal healthcare can be serviced by advice from the best physicians in the country—at home.
3. *Environmental and economic disasters and dislocations.* The prospect of natural and human-made disasters is growing through the pressures of population increases, urbanization, exhaustion of natural resources, and nuclear weapons. Witness the furor over the discovery of dioxin waste contamination in Times Beach, MO. This has serious healthcare consequences.
4. *Personal values and lifestyle.* Americans are showing increasing interest in simplicity, nutrition, exercise, "wellness" programs, and holistic approaches to health.
5. *New healthcare providers.* Americans are shifting from sole reliance on licensed physicians to wider accep-tance of licensed (or unlicensed) nonphysician health-care providers such as nurse-practitioners, midwives, dental hygienists, alternative therapists, and other

paraprofessional medical practitioners. These five, and other, "emerging issues" are part of the context within which future healthcare ministry will be exercised.[11]

The Content

As U.S. Catholic healthcare ministry moves into the future, what guides it? What is the *content* of the vision that attracts, propels, and directs? Many answers might be given to this very serious question. In this chapter I want to emphasize, as one primary component of that vision, the concept—the action—of *social justice.* I emphasize this relying on the constant positions CHA has taken reminding its membership that Catholic healthcare facilities must be committed to implementing the teachings of the church's social encyclicals, the spirit of the Second Vatican Council, and the call of the 1971 synod of bishops, which stated that "action on behalf of justice and participation in the transformation of the world...[are] a constitutive dimension of the preaching of the Gospel."[12]

How is social justice defined? It is the structuring of society so that institutions and social processes respect human dignity, protect human rights, and promote human development. Social justice is primarily a structural, rather than a personal, matter. It relates to the social structures of business, law, politics, trade unions, education, health, and church. We promote social justice not simply by personal charity or service, but by working for the structural transformation necessary to foster the dignity, rights, and development of all women and men. As the 1981 pastoral letter, *Health and Health Care,* states:

> The works of justice require that Christians involve themselves in sustained struggle to correct any unjust social, political, and economic structures and institutions which are the causes of suffering . . . . Because we believe in the dignity of the person, we must embrace every chance to help and to liberate, to heal the wounded of the world as Jesus taught us. Our hands must be the strong, but gentle hands of Christ, reaching out in mercy and justice, touching individual persons, but also touching the social conditions

that hinder the wholeness which is God's desire for humanity.[13]

CHA has identified five guidelines for taking practical steps to advance the cause of social justice: (1) set social justice goals; (2) establish just policies (e.g., relating to employment, discrimination); (3) promote social justice education; (4) promote social justice advocacy (e.g., relating to legislation); and (5) review investment policies. All these comprise the *content* of the vision moving Catholic healthcare ministry into the future. I would like to expand the understanding of that content, however, by briefly outlining seven themes that for me have both a *prominence* in church social teaching and a *relevance* in healthcare ministry.

1. *Human dignity.* This is the primary social teaching, on which everything else builds. The dignity of the person, of course, provides the check, the tool of evaluation, regarding all medical practices, such as the introduction of new technologies and the basic life-support decisions.

2. *Rights.* Flowing from the dignity of persons in society are human rights. Twenty years ago, in *Pacem in Terris,* Pope John XXIII outlined the basic rights of every person—legal and political, social and economic (echoing the Two Covenants of the United Nation's Universal Declaration of Human Rights).[14] On the pope's list was the basic right to medical care.[15] At the end of March 1983, the President's Commission for the Study of Ethical Problems in Medicine and Biomedical and Behavioral Research (chaired by Morris Abrams, former President of Brandeis University) concluded that society at large has an ethical obligation to ensure equitable access to healthcare for all citizens. The increasingly complex issue of access is an issue of rights.

3. *Participation.* The church's social teaching stresses the rights of people to have a say in decisions that affect them. I believe we need, for example, to examine the composition of boards of directors of Catholic healthcare facilities to see if these boards reflect participation by employees, patients, and community representatives (including the poor).

4. *The option for the poor.* From Latin America has come the renewed emphasis on the ancient Christian tradition—rooted in the teaching and example of Jesus and in the prophets of the Jewish scriptures—of giving a "preferential but non-exclusive option for the poor."[16] This provides us with a fundamental criterion for evaluating any plan or policy of a Catholic healthcare facility: what is happening to the poor? Obviously, we are *not* moving into a future guided by Catholic principles if our health facilities—in organization, operation, or orientation—are pulling away from service of the poor. This is most especially true because Catholic healthcare ministry in the United States was founded primarily to meet the needs of the poor.

5. *Workers.* From *On the Condition of Labor (Rerum Novarum)* in 1891 to *On Human Work (Laborem Exercens)* in 1981, Catholic social teaching has repeated the right of workers to organize into unions and to bargain collectively with management. The CHA's prize-winning book, *Issues in the Labor-Management Dialogue,* demonstrates both the continued centrality and the continued complexity of this issue.[17] I would simply comment that the healthcare ministry's future existence as well as future credibility of the church's overall social stance will depend very much on how CHA's membership accepts and implements this church teaching.[18]

6. *Social order.* "Holistic" is a good adjective to describe the social teaching's perspective on society. Economics, politics, and culture are closely interrelated in this perspective. Hence healthcare, ministering to the whole person, must take account of the total environment within which the person lives.[19]

7. *Common good.* A basic tenet of the church's social teaching, echoing the teaching of Thomas Aquinas, has always been the importance of the common good—that set of conditions wherein individual persons can achieve full humanity. A public authority, the government, is necessary to coordinate efforts to

promote the common good. In Christian political thought, then, the government is not seen as a minimal entity, a necessary evil, a thing to be feared. As our healthcare ministry relates increasingly to government in the future, this is an important point to keep in mind.

These seven themes are fundamental to the social justice content that guides the future of Catholic healthcare ministry.

I do acknowledge, however, that many people find it difficult to hear and believe the church's social teaching in the face of injustices within the church itself. The 1971 synod of bishops pointed to this by stating that it recognized "that anyone who ventures to speak to people about justice must first be just in their eyes."[20] Justice disputes involving people such as Agnes Mary Mansour, Charles Curran, and Raymond Hunthausen—just to give three examples—are especially painful blocks to serious engagement in the church's justice ministry.

The Consequence

Looking to the Catholic challenge for the future of building a healthy society, we have reviewed some elements of the context of that future and probed some themes of content guiding us into that future. I now want to discuss briefly what I see to be the major consequence. I use the simple but profound word *alternatives* to point to what I feel is necessary to shape the future and build a healthy society. My remarks at this point are suggestive and impressionistic, but perhaps they will recall to your own thinking some discussions you have been in, some materials you have read, and even some dreams you have dreamed.

Let me be clear at the outset. To speak of alternatives is not to reject the past. Rather, it is to build on the past, recognizing that much of the recent past—which we live today—was itself quite likely to have been an alternative to an earlier past. This is called "rooted change," or a healthy respect for tradition, healthy enough to move beyond it when necessary. A bit of history is helpful at this point. When the Catholic healthcare ministry began in this country in the 1800s, it was largely *substitutional;* i.e., it filled in for what was lacking, attending to the needs of the poor and neglected. As the ministry flourished in the recent 1900s, it became more of a *parallel* service, moving alongside the public and private for-profit health-care that developed, spurred on by government social welfare policies. Now, as we move into the future, I suggest that the ministry must search for ways to become more of an *alternative* form of service—in faithfulness to its particular charism and open to the influence of specifically Christian values. The prominent note of the substitutional era was *charity;* of the parallel era, *efficiency* and *professionalism;* and of the alternative era, *justice.*[21]

Drawing on the work of some futurists in healthcare research (especially a Canadian, Trevor Hancock, MD), let me suggest a series of seven shifts that make up an approach to alternatives. You yourself can fill in additional details as I mention the shifts. Dr. Hancock labels the shifts a movement from the "hard health path" to the "soft health path," borrowing from the discussion/debate in energy circles about "hard energy paths" such as petroleum or nuclear and "soft energy paths" such as solar.[22]

The "hard health path," much of what we experience as the dominant approach today, emphasizes:

1. A medical model—seeing sickness as the main problem
2. Medical care—providing surgery, drugs, physical therapy
3. Cure—overcoming sickness
4. Individual oriented—seeing each person in isolation
5. A technological approach—using the latest technology
6. Physician centered—doctors as primary
7. Institution based—regarding hospitals as primary

By contrast, the "soft health path," an alternative approach promoted even now in increasingly widening circles, emphasizes:

1. A human ecology model—seeing wellness as the main challenge
2. Environment/lifestyle—using a more holistic appreciation

3. Prevention—using education, nutrition, and exercise to maintain health. Palliative—incorporating suffering and dying into the life process
4. Community oriented—treating persons in relationship to wider society
5. Human/personal approach—focusing on high-touch, with sensitivity to the spiritual dimensions of healing
6. Nonphysician inclusive—using para-professionals and all other "healers" in society
7. Community based—being out amid the people, attached to other community institutions (nonhealth) such as parishes.

This set of seven contrasting approaches highlights much of the current discussion on alternatives. When I recently reread the bishops' pastoral letter, *Health and Health Care,* I was surprised to come across a section explicitly mentioning many of these alternative approaches. The section is found under the heading Prophetic Role. The bishops say that an "important way of fulfilling the church's prophetic role in the healthcare field is the development of alternative models of healthcare."[23]

And so I ask if this is not a major consequence facing the Catholic healthcare ministry today: To be a prophetic ministry by being particularly sensitive to the poor and particularly creative in exploring alternatives that will more faithfully reflect the church's social teaching by more explicitly attending to social justice. I have recently come to translate the phrase "social justice" as "alternatives." I believe that this translation has profound meaning for the future of Catholic healthcare ministry.

Conclusion

Let me conclude by presenting to you some questions concerning commitment.

1. *Personal.* Where do you see yourself in the future of Catholic healthcare ministry? Do you honestly experience a vocation, a movement of the Spirit, to continue giving yourself to this ministry as it evolves in new and challenging forms?

2. *Professional.* How can you better prepare yourself for the future? What steps can you take to stay in touch with, or provide leadership for, the development of alternative/justice approaches?

3. *Corporate.* What is your institution, your corporation, your congregation, and your Catholic Health Association doing to promote this movement into the future? What more should you do?

These questions regarding commitment should serve as a basis for both personal and liturgical prayer. We seriously need the light and strength of the Holy Spirit if we, as individuals and as community, are going to meet the Catholic challenge for the future: building a healthy society.

Footnotes

1. This chapter is a revision of the Flanagan Memorial Lecture give by Peter J. Henriot, SJ at the annual assembly of the Catholic Health Association. It was published in *Hospital Progress* in September 1983.
2. *Health and Health Care,* National Conference of Catholic Bishops, *Origins,* Vol. 11, No. 25, Dec. 3, 1981, p. 397.
3. Vatican Council II, *Pastoral Constitution on the Church in the Modern World,* #77, quoted in *The Challenge of Peace: God's Promise and Our Response,* #1. U.S. Catholic Conference, Washington DC, 1983, p. 1.
4. The World Bank, *The World Bank Atlas 1986.* The World Bank, Washington, DC, 1986, p. 16.
5. Robert S. McNamara, "Address to the Board of Governors of the World Bank," The World Bank, Washington, DC, Sept. 30, 1980.
6. *Economic Justice for All: Pastoral Letter on Catholic Social Teaching and the U.S. Economy,* National Conference of Catholic Bishops, U.S. Catholic Conference, Washington, DC, 1986, #25.
7. *The World Bank Atlas 1986,* pp. 12-15.
8. Ruth Leger Sivard, *World Military and Social Expenditures 1986.* World Priorities, Washington DC, 1986, p. 5.
9. Karl Rahner, SJ, "Towards a Fundamental Theological Interpretation of Vatican II," *Theological Studies,* 1979, pp. 716-727.
10. Paul Starr, *The Social Transformation of American Medicine: The Rise of a Sovereign Profession and the Making of a Vast Industry.* Basic Books, New York, 1982, p. 379.
11. For a fuller discussion of these issues see Clement Bezold, Rick J. Carlson, and Jonathan C. Peck, *The Future of Work and Health.* Auburn House Publishing Co., Dover, MA, 1986.
12. Synod of Bishops, Second General Assembly, *Justice in the World,* Vatican Polyglot Press, Vatican City, 1971.
13. *Health and Health Care,* p. 398.
14. Pope John XXIII, *Pacem in Terris.* America Press, New York, 1963, #11-38.
15. *Pacem in Terris,* #11.

16. John Eagleson and Philip Scharper, eds., *Puebla and Beyond: Documentation and Commentary.* Orbis Books, Maryknoll, NY, 1979, p. 222. This is #733 in the final document issued by the bishops at the Puebla meeting.
17. *Issues in the Labor-Management Dialogue: Church Perspectives,* Adam J. Maida, ed., The Catholic Health Association of the United States, St. Louis, 1982.
18. For more on the issues of unions, see Chapter 8, "The Call for a Prophetic Healthcare System," and Chapter 9, "Unionization, The Call of the Chuch and the Catholic Healthcare Institution."
19. For more on this issue, see Chapter 6, "Diagnosis: Good Healthcare in a Holistic Environment."
20. *Justice in the World,* #40. This text is also quoted in the U.S. bishops' economic pastoral. See *Economic Justice for All: Pastoral Letter on Catholic Social Teaching and the U.S. Economy* #347.
21. For more on these themes see Chapter 8, "The Call for a Prophetic Healthcare System."
22. Drawn from an unpublished manuscript written by Trevor Hancock, MD.
23. *Health and Health Care,* p. 401.

Reflection Questions

1. In reflecting on the context of healthcare today, this chapter highlights global poverty, the arms race, the church's shifting sense of identity, and several emerging trends in healthcare itself.
   - Are there any other significant factors in the context that should be noted?
   - What are they?
   - How do they affect healthcare ministry?

2. The problems of the world, the church, and healthcare, which form the context this chapter describes, seem overwhelming. As people of faith, we believe that God is present in the midst of ambiguities and that God's Spirit moves in and through apparent contradictions.
   - What signs of hope do you perceive in your world, and in the church, in healthcare?

3. The chapter indicates that the long term solution to the problems stated can be obtained by promoting social justice, not only by direct acts of charity or service but also through necessary structural transformations.
   - What practical steps promoting social justice are being implemented in your healthcare institution or system?
   - What steps could and should be taken?
   - How can a consciousness about these practical aspects of social justice be raised?
   - What commitment are you prepared to make?

4. As models of private collective ownership, Catholic healthcare institutions could exhibit a unique character and exert significant influence in the communities in which they operate.
   - How might the influence of these institutions help to infuse the vision and values of Jesus into the public sphere? Be specific.

5. The chapter cites examples in which the church's actions seemingly contradict the justice it proclaims.
   - What can the leadership in healthcare do to ensure that its institutions operationalize the values the church proclaims?
   - What systems of feedback and evaluation can be employed to measure the existence of or movement toward a just order among employees and patients, and between managerial levels of the institution?

6. An institution's prophetic stance is expressed by its willingness to explore alternative delivery systems that reflect "the soft health path" of wellness, holistic prevention, community orientation, and personal focus.
   - What groups do you see actively exploring such alternatives?
   - How can we move from the large institutional settings of the present to the broader community settings suggested for the future?
   - What groups of committed people do you see who could experiment and move forward into such new settings?

II

Clarifying
Our Identity

Actions are guided and influenced not only
by the needs of the context (Chapter 1) but also
by the identity of the actors. What is the
identity of Catholic healthcare today? Of its
various systems and facilities?

As Augustine said in a different context centuries ago, I know what something is
until someone asks me to define it. The rapid
escalation of healthcare costs, the emergence
of competitive for-profit systems, the federal
government's efforts to contain the cost of
medical care by forcing it into the marketplace, and a variety of other factors have combined to force healthcare institutions to
streamline their operations. What is essential?
What belongs to Catholic healthcare's very
nature? Catholic healthcare institutions and
systems have been asked to define it—and
more: to renew and reshape it. They are struggling with the task.

Chapter 2 challenges the contemporary tendency to redefine healthcare
primarily in terms of an economically efficient industrial corporation. To identify itself
as "the healthcare industry" providing
"product lines" for potential "customers" is,

the chapter argues, dangerous to the sense of ministry that should be healthcare's soul.

Chapter 3 takes the discussion another step. Clarifying the identity of Catholic healthcare institutions and systems will require healthcare personnel to reflect on their experience. The experience of God's presence and call revealed in the daily processes of the healing ministry is the foundation for a true sense of identity that can give appropriate direction to developing and promoting policy. The challenge of defining and clarifying our identity goes to the heart of our faith.

· 2 ·

Catholic Healthcare:
Competing and Complementary Models[1]

Peter J. Henriot, SJ

I would like to begin this chapter by recalling two important events that occurred within a week of each other not too long ago and that set a context for my reflections. The first event, on Tuesday, Nov. 6, 1984, was the reelection of President Ronald Reagan to four more years in office. However we might have been involved politically, we can read that reelection as an affirmation by 60 percent of the voters that the country was going in the right direction. Sixty percent of those who voted seemed to need and desire four more years of what we had been getting, both domestically and internationally.

Sunday of that same week, Nov. 11, 1984, the U.S. Catholic bishops began their annual meeting in Washington, DC, by presenting the first draft of a new pastoral letter. The pastoral on the economy, a very long document, said that the U.S. economy should be judged on what it is doing to and for people, particularly the poor. When it is judged according to that criterion, the bishops went on, our economy is not moving in a morally acceptable fashion.

I do not want to pose those two events as simply contradictory, but I do want to offer them as the context within which we live. We are living in a period in which the majority of the country's voters said, "Stay the course." Church leaders have said, "If we stay the course, at least be aware that there are significant moral

19

issues that need to be addressed very sharply at local, national, and international levels." Since that week the pastoral letter has gone through three drafts and been promulgated with overwhelming support from the bishops. Despite a great deal of pressure from Reagan supporters, they did not yield in their position.

These two events, in a sense, frame the debate within church-related circles (such as religiously affiliated healthcare systems) about the examination of our basic institutions—a debate to which all Americans are being called. This debate requires continual examination of education, social services, parishes, and healthcare institutions.

In this chapter I will grapple with the question of how much people who are part of religiously affiliated healthcare institutions within the larger U.S. healthcare system are influenced by and are able to influence both national and church developments. I will touch on five points: (1) the *uncertainties* facing religiously affiliated healthcare today; (2) the *models* for future healthcare; (3) the *trends* toward a healthcare industry; (4) the *calls* toward a healthcare ministry; and (5) some of the *consequences* for future care at institutional and personal levels.

Uncertainties

The uncertainties facing religiously affiliated institutions can be posed as follows: What model of healthcare will be dominant in determining future priorities and shaping future decisions? My thesis is a simple one: It states that *Catholic healthcare efforts in the years ahead must move more effectively toward healthcare ministry and not healthcare industry if it is to survive, and, indeed, if it is to deserve to survive.* Providing healthcare is a form of service in and for the community even before it is a form of economic activity. I know that that traditional principle guides the major portion of what people in Catholic healthcare do. Care is to be provided for whoever needs it. Later administrators will worry about who pays for that care. We all worry quite a bit about who pays for that care, but that worry is a secondary consideration.

Two parables help illustrate this point. The first is the parable of the Good Samaritan, in which the immediate response was to critical need on the road side. The second parable is contemporary. Shown on television just a few years ago, *The Day After*

20

was a story about what might occur after a nuclear explosion. The central figure was a physician. He responded immediately to the people's needs. No one checked insurance eligibility before meeting the people's needs in such an emergency.

Healthcare, whether it is an emergency or a service to people in need, is first a form of service for a community before it is a form of economic activity. These are not exclusive, mutually contradictory emphases, however. One must be efficient to be effective. One must exist to serve. But what I am suggesting is: Where is the shaping or visioning priority? What sets the tone, the direction, the distinctive marks, the unique characteristics, and the criteria for decision making? I want to suggest as an approach two models that are "polar types," the *ministry* model and the *industry* model.

Models

You have probably heard the story of President Truman confronting his newly formed Council of Economic Advisors. He said that he wanted a one-armed economist to be on his council. Asked why, President Truman replied that whenever he asked for the advice of economists, they always said, "On the one hand, this; and on the other hand, that." He wanted them to be clear and to have one-handed answers! Similarly when a social scientist speaks about different models, these models are usually "polar types." We put a lot of things on one side and emphasize this, and then a lot of things on another side and emphasize that. But reality is actually a mix of both. With that caution, let me suggest two healthcare models: *healthcare ministry* and *healthcare industry.*

Under the model of *healthcare ministry* are at least four different emphases.

1. Christian ministry is the *service of persons* as individuals in community through a loving concern for their well-being in the fullest sense. Healthcare ministry emphasizes respect for the person's dignity. The person who enters into a healthcare system guided by the model of ministry is first and foremost treated as a human being with all the rights each person has and with all the respect for dignity that each person demands simply by being a human being.

21

2. In healthcare ministry, there is concern for the whole person. There is a *holistic approach*. The person is not treated as an organism with isolated problems but as a whole; not just a whole individual person, but as part of that whole that is the relationship to the wider community, to that person's family, to that person's work, and to that person's social situation. Ministry always has an element of wholeness and concern for the whole.

3. Because of its holistic approach, ministry takes very seriously a specific *focus on the spiritual*. There is a real appreciation that the person has a spiritual dimension. Therefore, in healthcare ministry the spiritual dimension receives special attention. This is not the "spiritual dimension" in narrow religious terms. It calls for full sensitivity to the spirit that moves within a person and that must be related to in the healing process.

4. Ministry has a special *preference for the poor*. Catholic healthcare institutions and systems are clearly working hard to be faithful to this characteristic. Several systems have issued studies on the issue,[2] and The Catholic Health Association's *No Room in the Marketplace* stands as a clear call to the nation to face the problems confronting us.[3]

A special preference for the poor must be a note of ministry because ministry is a continuation of God's loving concern for us and of Jesus' service in the context of today. Always there is in God and in Jesus a special preference for the poor. Therefore, ministry and the ministry model must have a preference for the poor.

The other approach to healthcare is the model of *healthcare industry*. Although the contrasts between the models of healthcare ministry and healthcare industry may not always be clear cut, it is important to try to get a sense of the differing major emphases. I suggest that the healthcare industry model has four contrasting emphases when compared with the healthcare ministry model.

1. Industry is organized to offer a product or a service through the *pursuit of profit*. An industry incorporated

for profit must by law focus on a return on investment. If stockholders' money is taken, it is taken as a trust or investment. This profit orientation is a primary entry point for understanding the industry model.

2. The industry model focuses on *specialization for efficiency*. Efficiency is necessary to have cost effectiveness, which promotes a better return on investment. This specialization approach requires breaking down activities and procedures into different components and focusing on individual parts rather than on the whole.

3. There is a special concentration on *technological effectiveness*. One of the consequences of specialization in contemporary scientific society is a strong emphasis on technologies to make the industry's organization and operation effective.

4. Because industry exists in an environment of economic survival, there is *competition* to pursue that return on investment. Ability to compete is a key criterion for survival, and maintaining a competitive edge is a primary goal.

Although these two models are clearly complementary—one must have some economic efficiency, for example, to be able to serve—they also compete violently at some important points. For example, the primacy of the person's dignity can conflict with the type of return on investment that can be made. In the current economic environment, we must not let the quality of care drop. There are too many pressures today to let the human person's dignity take second place to an "adequate" return on investment in programs we offer. Moreover, to really see the person in a holistic fashion sometimes conflicts with a model that emphasizes specialization. Someone takes care of my blood pressure. Someone else takes care of my heartbeat. Someone else takes care of my nutrition. Someone else takes care of my gallbladder. But who takes care of me as a whole person? Specialization is always a challenge to a holistic approach.

The technical and the technological, so very effective in meeting many of today's needs, can override or at least conflict with an appreciation of and attention to the spiritual. And because

23

the industry model must pay very strict attention to competition, it can easily forget those who hurt an institution's competitive position if it attends to their needs—the poor. There is indeed no room for the poor in the competitive marketplace. Table 1 compares the two models.

TABLE 1:
COMPETING AND COMPLEMENTARY MODELS

Ministry Model	Industry Model
Service of persons	Pursuit of profit
Holistic approach	Specialization for efficiency
Focus on spiritual	Technological effectiveness
Preference for the poor	Competition for survival

We must ask: Which type, which model, guides the basic thrust of the decisions we are making? When people know a Catholic healthcare institution or system, is the first thing they associate with it service of the human person in a holistic approach that focuses on the spiritual and shows a preference for the poor? Then they are able to say: "That is a ministry. The people who work for that institution are drawn not to a job, but are called to a ministry."

Trends

My third point concerns some of the trends that reinforce an industry model in healthcare. The "medical-industrial complex," as *Newsweek* highlighted in a cover story several years ago, is the dominant fact of healthcare today.[4] Paul Starr, the Harvard professor who authored the major study on the social transformation of American medicine, highlighted this industrial development as the most influential factor in healthcare in the United States.[5] Medicine has indeed become a very large business—one of the largest employers in the economy, accounting for over 10 percent of the Gross National Product (GNP).

The movement toward a "healthcare industry" mentality is reflected in a very simple way in the language used: corporations, systems, chief executive officer, systems analysis, marketing, consumers, strategic planning, delivery systems, cost effectiveness, competition, growth. These phrases, all taken from recent Catholic healthcare documents, have become commonplace. It is important to remember, however that language shapes reality as well as reflects it. The more we use such language, the more we create a "healthcare industry" mentality.

As we discern trends reinforcing certain models, it is important to examine our language. Could contemporary healthcare ministry be carried on with a different vocabulary? Catholic healthcare might very well distinguish itself from the rest of healthcare and from the domination of society at large by business interests by changing its language. It would be a clear sign that Catholic healthcare wants to distinguish itself by offering healthcare *ministry* as its primary focus. The question is: Is our language in some sense letting us assume as a primary model a model that we do not in fact hold as primary?

I would like to mention seven factors promoting a concentration on healthcare as *industry*.

1. The first factor that pushes us toward an industry model is the growing expense of healthcare services. In 1986 the figure was $460 billion out of the U.S.'s $4.2 trillion GNP—about 11 percent.[6] Per capita annual healthcare expenses for every man, woman, and child in the United States, therefore, run around $1,900. In 1966 it was $129. In 1983 the increase of healthcare expenses slowed for the first time in a decade, rising only 10.3 percent; from 1972 to 1982 the average increase had been around 13 percent. The growth in the GNP from 1973 to 1983 averaged only 2.4 percent. Healthcare expenses are rising much faster than ordinary expenses and the GNP.

   A variety of explanations account for this increase. The American Medical Association (AMA) has urged physicians to refrain from raising fees as one way to curb rising expense. The government is using diagnosis-related groups (DRGs) to contain medical costs. Even the satirists are attacking the problem: Art Buchwald has proposed an "operation of the month" club, similar in format to the Book of the Month Club.

2. The rapid rise of for-profit healthcare systems now accounts for about 15 percent of all healthcare facilities, with revenues of over $10 billion. And these large corporations are becoming even larger. We can expect some multinational corporations to move into this area. For-profit institutions operate the newer and better facilities, although they do charge more and increase overall healthcare expenses. They are also moving into university-operated hospitals, a move that tends to promote the industry model in healthcare.

3. The question of access to resources and services is yet another element. In reality we may already have a two-tiered system in this country. A special Presidential Commission examining healthcare a few years ago cited as a serious danger the contrast between those who can pay or have good insurance programs and those who cannot pay and do not have any programs. CHA's study, *No Room in the Marketplace,* described some of the shocking contrasts in service that it discovered.[7]

4. Then there is the influence of expensive new technologies. Marvelous new methods are being developed rapidly, but they are also creating problems of expense and resource allocation. The purchase of the newest generation of computed tomography (CT) scanner influences the whole budget. Frequently physicians will order tests with the new technologies to safeguard themselves against the rising threat of malpractice suits. New technologies, of course, also raise a variety of ethical issues around life support.

5. New technologies will also influence who is employed within a hospital. One recent study estimated that by the year 2000 the staff portion of healthcare will be cut by 15 to 20 percent because of newly automated equipment, computers, and robots. These staff cuts would come in housekeeping, food services, laundry, maintenance, and accounting.

6. Changing attitudes of healthcare professionals, questions of physicians' status and their concern about the increasing cost of malpractice insurance, the public's changing expectations about the need for better healthcare (a new mood and a new movement, more personal concern, diet, exercising)—all these factors push in the direction of the industry model. Declining censuses can be accounted for by a variety of factors, but certainly one of the key factors is "consumers'" new attitudes.

7. An expanded government role and influence in a variety of areas is also a major factor affecting the future of healthcare. The experience of DRGs clearly bears this out.

Calls

In briefly sketching this healthcare environment, I suggest that these influences push us more and more toward the industry model. But what calls us toward the ministry model? What provides a balance? Ministry obviously continues to be the ideal of religiously affiliated health institutions. Although it is true that such institutions often use the language of the corporate world when expressing their mission, they also use language that conveys a sense of ministry. Mission statements often express a call to be faithful to the spirit of the sponsoring congregation and to witness to the love of Jesus and his Creator for all people through health services that promote community, advance the quality of life, revere dignity in death, and respond to all people's unmet health needs in a rapidly changing world. This type of vision is a powerful expression of the ministry model.

The emphasis on ministry in healthcare comes from a variety of sources, just as the emphasis on an industry model does. It is helpful to be aware of them. Four of them are the tradition, the charisms, the teachings, and the expectations.

1. The traditional understanding of healthcare emphasizes service. Again and again, no matter where people are within the system or how they have come into that system, the call to service is there to prod them. Healthcare incorporates a call to service; it should

never be viewed primarily as an economic activity. The tradition from the very beginning is that *healthcare ministers to people.* Even under siege, that tradition lives on.

2. This tradition has been highlighted and captured in the charisms or special characteristics of the congregations that founded religiously affiliated institutions. The congregations have invited others to share in that ministry, to be enriched by sharing in it, and in turn to enrich the understanding of what that ministry is about. The charism is a strong call to keep the ministry model paramount.

3. Church teachings help shape the vision of the religiously affiliated healthcare systems. The U.S. bishops' pastoral letter on the economy discusses what has been called "the best kept secret in the Catholic church," its social teaching.[8] The clearest lesson of that teaching is that what goes on in society—economically, politically, socially, culturally—is not religiously neutral; it is central to whether the Reign of God comes alive in our midst. It is church teaching that through ministry the efforts and the continuation of God's Reign go on and Jesus' presence is felt.[9]

In their pastoral letter *Health and Health Care,* the U.S. bishops stated the call more specifically: "Members of the church follow the example of Jesus when they carry out the work of healing, not only by providing care for the physically ill, but also by working to restore health and wholeness in all facets of the human person and the human community."[10]

4. The call for ministry comes from the expectations of the larger community—the Catholic community, the Christian community, the civil community—that over the years has supported the Catholic healthcare system. People do expect that a religiously affiliated institution will be different. It is not simply the crucifix in a hospital room, or prayers over a loudspeaker, or sisters who move about, or the availability of a hospital chapel. It is something more: healthcare according to the ministry model.

Special attention should be paid within the ministry model to the call for concern for the poor. The church has called this special concern "the preferential but non-exclusive option for the poor." I suggest that we reflect for a moment on this preferential option.

One way of attempting to live out that option already marks many healthcare institutions and systems significantly by their *direct* provision of services for those who cannot pay, by not turning people away, by reaching out directly to people in need. But there is also a very important *indirect* way in which institutions exercise their option for the poor. This involves working to affect overall national policy concerning the poor. Healthcare systems are major societal actors—not just in the services they offer directly to the poor but also in the actions they undertake to bring about institutional change in society.[11]

For example, the treatment offered to employees within the healthcare system should be a model for the rest of society of treatment that respects human dignity and the poor. The difficult question of unionization in hospitals is an important instance of this issue. The bishops' letter on the economy puts it very clearly: no one is going to believe the Catholic church when it talks about justice in the economy unless it is just in its own economic operations.[12] How we grapple with employees' rights to organize into unions will be an important test of whether we are authentically in the ministry model and whether our call for justice in the wider society will have any credibility.

Public stances made by the healthcare institutions represent another indirect way of responding to the option for the poor. What are Catholic healthcare systems known for as they relate to different public policies in healthcare—for example, national health insurance, Medicaid and Medicare problems, the government's cutbacks? Do the systems opt for the poor in the public stances they take? At the local level, what type of presence and influence do they exert in the community? For instance, the people who serve on the board of trustees should be invited into a ministerial role in the local community. They should represent—in their business practices, in their educational outlooks, in the way they raise their families—a ministerial stance that takes very seriously the issue of the poor in our society today. What I want to emphasize here is that if we reduce the option for the poor simply to direct service for the poor, we miss some of the major challenges before us for shaping our society for the future.

Another issue that deserves a great deal of attention today is the matter of *alternatives*. Can Catholic institutions offer an arena for showing that alternative approaches to healthcare— healthcare education, holistic health approaches, community-based healthcare, participation in healthcare—are central and not peripheral? These topics have been discussed for many years. I believe that religiously affiliated healthcare institutions and systems committed to the ministry model are the best places to experiment with alternative approaches.[13]

Consequences

Finally, I want to consider some of the consequences of these reflections on healthcare ministry for the future of health-care. Times are changing very rapidly. We must be sensitive to the potential consequences of our choices.

First, healthcare institutions and systems must shape realistic mission statements. They must recognize that a tension will exist between the two models. The title of this chapter is "Catholic Healthcare: Competing and Complementary Models." The two models are indeed complementary—institutions must exist to serve. But they are also competing. Any mission statement must be explicit and realistic. It must indicate clearly that the primary model governing the institution is the healthcare ministry model.

That step will affect a number of things. For instance, it will set into place continual evaluation of local and board decisions—an evaluation based on the principles of the ministry model. Whatever decision is made—to open or close an institution, to hire a person, to move in a particular direction—the basic question for evaluation will be: How does this serve ministry? It is not the only question to ask, but it is the primary question. This has implications for recruitment criteria. Persons should be hired not just on the basis of their technical skills, but because, in a genuine sense, they share the values we want to promote. There should be a continual effort in hiring and promotion to see that employees are committed to ministry values.

Training programs, then, should be central. There must be a continual helping of everyone at every level—medical staff, trustees, house maintenance staff, nurses—to understand the particular charism that founded this institution as a form of ministry and that continues the institution as ministry. That will require ongoing in-service training, not only about the sponsor's charism but also about church social teaching and relevant moral and ethical issues.

Let me make a concrete suggestion. It would be exciting if all U.S. Catholic healthcare institutions took as part of their in-service training for the next few months the document of the bishops on the economy. Trustees, medical staff, administrators, and employees should grapple with this document and the ethical concerns it raises. What marks a healthcare system that emphasizes ministry is that its ethical concerns are not only *microethical*. They are also *macroethical*. Microethical issues—i.e., more personal issues such as sterilization and maintenance of life—are important, but equally important and unfortunately not attended to by many Catholic ethicists, are the macroethical issues of access to adequate healthcare for all, treatment of the poor, rootedness in community, and plans for the future.

Finally, I want to say a word about "vocation." One of the primary consequences of an emphasis on the ministry model is the need to discern one's vocation. It is a challenge for all who are involved in healthcare: Why are we drawn to this work? Do we feel called to it? Is it truly a vocational commitment? Whatever our religious background might be, we all understand that there is a difference between going to a job and being called to a ministry. The ministry model will never stay alive unless it is nurtured by people who feel a call.

Conclusion

I conclude by returning to the U.S. bishops' pastoral letter on the economy. In the second and fourth chapters of that document, the bishops issue a call for a "New American Experiment."[14] They remind us that many of our ancestors came to this country to escape the morally unacceptable conditions of political deprivation and persecution that they had experienced. Our country was born as an experiment in political democracy,

31

with people cooperating together to promote the rights and well-being of all.

Today, according to the pastoral, there are morally unacceptable conditions of economic deprivation: high levels of unemployment, great gaps between rich and poor, hunger in this nation and around the world, and so on. It is time to commit ourselves as a nation to recognizing economic rights—including the right to adequate healthcare—as authentic human rights due all people.[15] And we must experiment with economic democracy, with all people cooperating together to promote the rights and well-being of all through such mechanisms as cooperatives, worker ownership and worker-management schemes, revitalized unions, plant-closing legislation and provision for re-training, and new forms of local, regional, national, and international economic cooperation.[16]

Some very challenging opportunities lie before us as we struggle to meet this nation's healthcare needs. By scrutinizing the complementary and competing models of healthcare ministry and healthcare industry, we will contribute not only to a healthy health-care system but to a healthy nation. And that is a very exciting project indeed.

Footnotes

1. This chapter is a revision of an address first given to the Holy Cross Health System.
2. To give just a few examples: Holy Cross Health System, *1983 System Report* highlighting "The Needy Shall Not Be Forgotten"; Bon Secours Health System, *Bon Secours Means Good Help To Those In Need: Report and Recommendations of the Bon Secours Task Force on the Care of the Poor,* August 1985; and Sisters of Mercy Health Corporation, *Health Services For the Poor: A Challenge to Public Policy,* 1985.
3. *No Room in the Marketplace: Health Care of the Poor,* The Catholic Health Association of the United States, St. Louis, 1986. This is the final report of CHA's Task Force on Health Care of the Poor as approved by the CHA Board of Trustees on April 24, 1986.
4. "The Big Business of Medicine," *Newsweek,* Oct. 31, 1983, pp. 62-74.
5. Paul Starr, *The Social Transformation of American Medicine: The Rise of a Sovereign Profession and the Making of a Vast Industry.* Basic Books, New York, 1982, pp. 200-206, 315-318, 420-449. See especially pp. 428-429.
6. Maureen Dowd, "U.S. Health Care Faulted in Senate," *The New York Times,* Jan. 13, 1987, pp. A1, B7.
7. "In stark contrast to the frustration, pain, and even death endured by many sick and uninsured poor persons, a recent news article reveals how some U.S. hospitals have begun to compete for affluent patients by offering luxury suites and hot tubs. The article cites a wealthy patient's experience in a large

Midwestern hospital. The patient invited a friend to dinner in his hospital room. They began with appetizers of herring and pickled vegetables and then moved on to chateaubriand. After dinner they watched *Amadeus* on [the patient's] large screen television set . . . .'The hospital's room service was just as nice as a fancy hotel,' [the patient said] . . 'and the room looked like a high-rise luxury apartment.'" *No Room in the Marketplace: Health Care of the Poor.* The Catholic Health Association of the United States, St. Louis, 1986, p. 4.

8. *Economic Justice for All: Pastoral Letter on Catholic Social Teaching and the U.S. Economy,* National Conference of Catholic Bishops, U.S. Catholic Conference, Washington, DC, 1986, Chapter 2. For a brief synopsis of most of the major documents of Catholic social teaching, see Peter J. Henriot, Edward P. DeBerri, and Michael J. Schultheis, *Catholic Social Teaching: Our Best Kept Secret,* Center of Concern/Orbis Books, Maryknoll, NY, 1988.

9. "Christian communities that commit themselves to solidarity with those suffering and to confrontation with those attitudes and ways of acting which institutionalize injustice will themselves experience the power and presence of Christ." *Economic Justice for All: Pastoral Letter on Catholic Social Teaching and the U.S. Economy,* #55.

10. *Health and Health Care,* National Conference of Catholic Bishops, *Origins,* Vol. 11, No. 25, Dec. 3, 1981, p. 397.

11. I have developed some of these thoughts further in Chapter 5, "Service of the Poor: The Foundation of Judeo-Christian Response." This is a revision of an essay entitled "Service of the Poor: A Basis for Spirituality and Mission" in *Justice and Health Care,* Sr. Margaret John Kelly, ed., The Catholic Health Association of the United States, St. Louis, 1985, pp. 13-29.

12. *Economic Justice for All: Pastoral Letter on Catholic Social Teaching and the U.S. Economy,* #347.

13. For more on this, see Chapter 1, "Building a Healthy Society: A Catholic Challenge of the Future."

14. *Economic Justice for All: Pastoral Letter on Catholic Social Teaching and the U.S. Economy,* #95, #295-325.

15. *Economic Justice for All: Pastoral Letter on Catholic Social Teaching and the U.S. Economy,* #79-95.

16. *Economic Justice for All: Pastoral Letter on Catholic Social Teaching and the U.S. Economy,* #295-325.

Reflection Questions

1. What shapes the direction, the distinctive marks, and the unique characteristics for decision making in your healthcare setting?
   - Can you identify a shaping or visionary priority?
   - What model, the ministry or industry, prevails? Explain the reasons your answer. Give examples.

2. This chapter suggests the following characteristics as identifying marks of the healthcare ministry model: focused on the *human person* in a *holistic way* that emphasizes the *spiritual* and shows *a preference for the poor.*
   - Do these marks describe your service, your institution(s)?
   - Must you take exception to any of the above?
   - How can current operations be changed to model these marks so that they would incorporate these characteristics?

3. The industry model of healthcare leaves no room for the care of the poor and the uninsured. The chapter suggests that exercising the church's preferential option for the poor is one way an institution witnesses to the ministry model. This option can be exercised through direct service to the poor or through action on their behalf.
   - Does a preferential option for the poor influence decision making in your establishment? How?
   - Are you aware of any indirect efforts in which your institution is engaged, or which your institution supports, that promote structural and institutional changes in favor of the poor?

4. This chapter couches the economics of healthcare within the context of the 1986 social statement of the U.S. bishops, *Economic Justice for All.*
   - Have you read this document? If not, how might you become familiar with it?
   - What first steps would you suggest that might lead to this document's principles being internalized by those persons who shape decisions that affect your establishment economically?

5. Trials reveal what lies hidden in the human heart. God speaks
    to each generation in a language they can understand to lead
    human beings to a deeper vision of the divine designs of peace
    and love. From this moment of crisis in healthcare, God can
    extract a new starting point. The chapter suggests we experi-
    ment with economic democracy.
    - How would you suggest we do this?
    - Do you think all people can cooperate to promote the
      common good?
    - How might you experiment with more worker management
      or forms of worker ownership in your institution(s)?

· 3 ·

Shaping Public Policy: A Challenge in Faith[1]

James E. Hug, SJ

This is a crucial time for religiously grounded not-for-profit health-care facilities and systems. They are being asked to play an increasingly active role in shaping public policy. At the same time, the U.S. courts have consistently reaffirmed the separation of church and state by disallowing even a moment of silence for prayer in public schools. The most political pope in recent history insists that the church stay out of politics. The bishops have stirred major debate by speaking out on nuclear arms policy and the U.S. economy. A Mercy sister, Agnes Mary Mansour, underwent a painful ecclesiastical procedure because she pursued the political call of her Mercy vocation.

Looking at that turmoil, healthcare administrators may say to themselves, "Who needs it! Our service is healing, comforting. We do it well. We should be doing it even better. Leave public policy issues to the politicians." But the question is no longer *whether* healthcare professionals will be involved in public policy, but *how* they will be involved. If they attempt to stay out of public policy debate, they automatically serve and support present policies. The religious healthcare community's size and organization give it a power that cannot be ignored. Those most deeply involved in the healthcare ministry must reflect on its religious dimensions to determine what guidance these dimensions might offer for public policy.[2]

36

More important than the practical aspect of involvement in public policy is the moral and religious imperative that is central to the identity of healers in the Judeo-Christian tradition. In the 1971 synod document *Justice in the World,* bishops from around the world affirmed a growing recognition in the church that work for social justice is a constitutive part of the Gospel.[3] It is not a voluntary good work. It is not something to be added to one's principal work if he or she has time and energy. It is an essential part of Christian life.

Contemplating that insight, we realize that it demands rethinking our Christian vocations. We need, for example, a new sense of what it means to be a Catholic healthcare facility in the Judeo-Christian tradition—a facility that addresses the issues embedded in the mesh of intertwined socioeconomic structures, social networks, and institutions in the global society of which we are all a part. As healthcare personnel know well, when they reach out to heal and comfort in a spirit of mercy, dozens of federal, state, and local programs and regulations try to direct their touch—not to mention the institutional and church policies or the larger social policy contexts that shape healthcare.[4] Sometimes these programs and regulations help; sometimes they do not. Sometimes they seem designed to exclude those most in need. And sometimes they waste precious resources.[5]

Anyone hoping to carry out a ministry of healing must work to heal the nation's social structures (and the church's as well). Bureaucratic and socioeconomic injustices generated by healthcare systems must be challenged. The national consciousness must be called to assume attitudes of healing concern. Otherwise, society will continue to spawn diseases, such as those rooted in poverty, malnutrition, and nuclear radiation, to which healthcare professionals and institutions must respond.

It is unnecessary to identify here the specific areas of healthcare policy demanding attention. This discussion will consider instead the faith reflection that is needed to guide public policy involvement.

Public Policy and Religious Belief

The recession of the early 1980s and the country's general economic history during the past 10 years have forced us

37

to analyze deeply what we believe and value. The national commitment to healthcare as a human right, made at a time of peak economic development in the 1960s, has been affected by the actions of oil-producing countries, a deepening cold war-style arms race, and mushrooming federal deficits. That commitment today suffers seriously from severe cutbacks in medical funds. The Colorado state legislature, for example, enacted a law stating that medically indigent are not entitled to medical services as a matter of right.[6]

Some see current trends as a reneging on the Judeo-Christian commitment to the poor, aged, and needy. I am sympathetic to their perspective, but the public policy debate is considerably more complex. And, strangely enough, it is being recognized increasingly as, in significant part, a theological debate.

Public policies are rooted—usually unconsciously—in religious beliefs, and religious beliefs have social and political dimensions. Formal mission statements of religiously affiliated healthcare institutions and systems usually begin as follows:

> Inspired by Christ Jesus and by the example of our foundress/founder, we of the _____
> Health Corporation, participating in the healing mission of the Catholic church, affirm our commitment to serve our community—especially the needy, the ill, the disabled. In our works we affirm the dignity and value of each person. Within the limits of our resources we dedicate our efforts to aid all persons in their striving for human wholeness—physically, spiritually, socially, and intellectually.

The members of that healthcare system are called to work for recognition of the right of all to necessary healthcare, compassionate service, and a social situation that promotes health. In this context, the Reagan Administration's cuts in social programs represented moves in exactly the wrong direction.

In recent years, Christians who favor the administration's policies—or who generally tend to support conservative political policies—have begun to speak out against the churches' liberal social positions. "We, too," they say, "believe in Jesus Christ and try to live our lives by his inspiration. We too," they might continue, "find the various foundresses and founders of religious healthcare institutions inspiring persons. We consider ourselves involved participants in the church's healing mission. But more social programs are not the answer. They are dangerous and irresponsible. Reagan's agenda is the answer—and we are not less Christians for saying so!'"[7]

These persons are attempting to work out the religious reasons for their policy positions and thus challenging all parties involved to do the same. The tensions that arise are not unknown in the boardrooms of Catholic institutions when business people and religious professionals sit down together to set policy. A brief review of three different theological approaches may help to indicate the type of further theological reflection needed and help reconcile some of these basic differences.[8]

Theology of Democratic Capitalism

The theology of democratic capitalism received public attention in the early 1980s, most of it associated with Michael Novak, who succeeded generally in articulating the business community's spirit and vision and received from it a great deal of support in return. Other voices have helped develop the theology of democratic capitalism, but, for the purposes of this discussion, Novak can serve as spokesperson.[9]

He sums up much of his thought in this paragraph:
To look upon history as love-infused by a Creator who values others as others, who sees in those originating sources of insight and choice which we have come to know as "persons" the purpose of [God's] creation; and who in loving each as an individual creates of the contrarious many an unseen, hidden, but powerful community, is to glimpse a world in which the political economy of democratic capitalism makes sense.[10]

Novak's metaphor for God is important: God is the Creator. The creation, he explains, is an evolutionary process characterized by ever-shifting forces that open up new possibilities. No single, static plan details the ordering of things—not even God's mind. God is the practical, ever-adapting creative genius.

Creation's central value is the human person. Each individual is called to be a free, creative source of insight and choice. True Christian love is like God's love: a love that respects others' freedom. That type of love best serves the common good. To set out consciously to promote the common good is to risk imposing someone's ideals on others. That has the double evil effect of suppressing creative freedom and creating dependencies. From this perspective, social programs may be well intentioned; but if they unnecessarily limit individual human freedom either directly or indirectly, they cannot claim to reflect God's will.

The greatest evil is the oppressive use of power to impose on other persons' freedom. Democratic capitalism is praised as a system of political economy because it is organized to prevent the centralization of power. Democratic capitalism protects against governments' potential tyranny by diffusing power in society. The economic realm is separated from the political and thrives on the competition of creative individuals. Competition diffuses power in society and brings out its members' creative potential. That is why free-market capitalism has proved so productive.

Since it is clear that gifts and talents are not distributed equally, Novak concludes that equality is of limited concern to God. God's purpose in creation is the free, creative individual. Each individual's freedom of choice must be protected—and for that, an approximate equality of opportunity is important. Justice should be seen by Christians, Novak argues, as equality of opportunity and as responsible stewardship of creation's productive capabilities. Competition in the free marketplace protects these in most cases. Where it fails, however, the state should have enough power to reinstate it—but no more.

The way in which democratic capitalism reflects the Creator's will and activity and protects against tyranny justifies its defense at almost any cost. The Soviet brand of socialism, for example, uses highly centralized government power to suppress its people's freedom. Although Novak disclaims the position personally, it seems coherent with the theological perspective of democratic capitalism to support President Reagan's assessment of it as an "evil empire."[11] We must arm to prevent its spread. It seems only logical too that the country's healthcare system should be prepared to cooperate with government contingency plans in case of nuclear attack, although Novak insists that in a pluralistic society it cannot be coerced into doing so.

In this context, it is not just idealistic to speak of needed healthcare as a basic human right.[12] It is dangerously utopian and practically immoral. It waters down the notion of humans and raises people's hopes and expectations beyond what society's wealth can provide. It is sure to create the social frustration that leads to political pressure to expand federal programs, thereby increasing government's power.

Such government programs tend to instill dependencies. They remove the incentive for creativity and hard work, which not only bring healthcare within individuals' and families' economic reach but enrich everyone in the process. By increasing taxes to finance them, such programs remove the incentive of the wealthy and the middle class to produce. Since these are, when left to themselves, the most productive sectors in society, this is an especially serious matter. As cocreators with God, we have the responsibility, Novak argues, to act more wisely.

The focus of policy guidance from democratic capitalism is clear. Although equality of opportunity is to be sought as realistically as possible and some social safety net is undoubtedly necessary, we should be wary of social programs. They should be left as much as possible to individual initiative in the private sector, evoking human creativity—not to mention charity—in the Creator's image rather than promoting dependencies.

The principles outlined here can be extended to the healthcare industry as well. Those who express concern about the development of for-profit healthcare systems[13] should rest assured, or even join the trend. Competition will make the industry more productive and help reduce costs. If unequal availability of healthcare results, that should not cause great concern, since equality of results does not seem to be important to the Creator.[14]

Furthermore, that inequality can be an incentive for the poor to expend greater effort to provide for their families and loved ones. Operating healthcare facilities with good business sense leaves everyone better off than if administrators and boards of directors pursue policies arising from a naive (albeit well-intentioned) compassion.

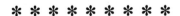

41

By now I hope I have been able to clarify how basic experiences of God are related to and support social policies. One's fundamental sense of God sheds light on the meaning and purpose of human life and, therefore, on the type of social policies necessary to support and promote it. Although Novak's argument is narrow and weak, it is a theological argument and calls for a theological response. It urges us to ask, What is *our* experience of God? What is *our* sense of healing mission? What guidance do *they* give for shaping public policy?

Theology of Stewardship

A strikingly different theological perspective on economic issues appeared in the United States in the late 1970s. A number of people concerned with world hunger and the availability of natural resources began to organize their reflections around the biblical notion of *stewardship*.[15] Their work is available in a book called *The Earth is the Lord's: Essays on Stewardship*.[16]

This topic was selected by The Catholic Health Association of the United States as the theme of its Twelfth Annual Catholic Health Assembly in 1983. As a result, it was also the subject of a number of articles and news reports in *Hospital Progress* during 1983. The dominance of this theological motif in the reflection of the religious healthcare community makes it an appropriate and important example here.

The primary religious experience shaping stewardship theology is the felt sense of God's goodness and love in creation. All creation is God's wonderful gift, entrusted to us, to all humanity. Love is, as the first letter of John says, God loving us first.[17] We are God's image entrusted with creation. As we contemplate the gift of it all, we feel deep appreciation and awe. Gratitude stirs within us a sense of obligation to respect creation and to care for it.

In this sense, no one really owns property; all are stewards of God's creation. The principal reason for the institution of private property, as St. Thomas Aquinas pointed out in the 13th century, is not that individuals have a right or absolute claim to it. Rather property, which belongs to everyone, is allotted to individuals so that better care will be taken of that part of the creation entrusted to us by God for all.[18]

Violating that trust—the root sin—can take many forms. For instance, assuming that property ownership is absolute and that others have no right to it—no matter what their need—is sinful.[19] The gap between the wealthy and the poor around the world bears shameful witness to this attitude. Lack of care for what has been entrusted to us is another form of sin, as is any oppression or injustice against our sisters and brothers.

Our calling is not simply to promote the development of more products and services through individual achievement in a competitive free market. That approach has proved destructive to both natural resources and human community. Rather, we must grow in gratitude for the gifts of creation, especially for every person within it. We must let ourselves become free enough to share in God's bias in favor of the weak and victimized, to share in Jesus' bias in favor of enemies and those in need, and to share in the Holy Spirit's bias in favor of hope. The scriptures show God on the side of the poor and oppressed, offering a vision of hope for a society based on gratitude, justice, and love.

In this context, justice is not defined as equality of opportunity. Justice calls for a distribution of goods and services based on need. Those who need healthcare should have it. It is proper to speak of a universal right to healthcare. The right to healthcare is grounded in God's gift of creation's resources to all. Cooperation and grateful sharing—not competition and private ownership—are primary characteristics of this Christian lifestyle.

Government programs that serve these goals are good. Government power used to steward wisely the resources of creation is not evil or dangerous. Efforts to reach out to all enemies in hope of reconciliation must be made. The contemporary arms race not only ignores the call to healing reconciliation, it wastes terribly the resources entrusted to us. Indeed, it threatens the very survival of human life on this planet.[20] Let the Pentagon hold fund-raising drives if it must, but invest tax monies to serve the world's sick, needy, and oppressed. The vocation to stewardship demands nothing less.

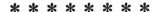

This faith reflection obviously sets out a quite different public policy direction than the first one I described. It has its strengths; it also has its weaknesses. Its importance here is that it, too, raises the questions: Who do *we* say God is? How do *we* know Jesus and his mission? How do *we* experience the call to the healing ministry? What guidance does that calling give *us* in public policy debate?

The answer is not to be found simply in choosing one or another of the options described. Although the general theme of stewardship promises to be more adequate and appropriate than the theology of democratic capitalism, both models are incomplete. I use them here to demonstrate the links between specific faith visions and public policy orientations. They should not be approached as ready-made theological commodities packaged to attract consumer choice. Their purpose is to spur personal and corporate faith reflection on life experience.

The U.S. Bishops' Pastoral Letter on Health and Healthcare

A third model is available in the U.S. bishops' 1981 pastoral letter, *Health and Healthcare*.[21] The letter reflects on Jesus' healing ministry, the biblical notion of health as personal and social wholeness, and the dignity of human persons as images of God to guide public policy development in healthcare. It underlines personal and familial responsibilities for health as well as public and private institutions' obligations. It calls for an ambitious program of social reform, including national health insurance.

The bishops' statement, however, remains a model. It must not replace personal theological reflection either, even though it is an official church document. The voices of those in healthcare must be heard. As Most Rev. James W. Malone, bishop of Youngstown, OH, indicated in addressing the Twelfth Catholic Health Assembly, the bishops need the healthcare professionals as active participants in forming the church's response to healthcare needs.[22] The most important revelation of the changes and developments needed in healthcare policy is given in the ordinary daily experience of those trying to heal as Jesus did. That revelation is manifested in the successes—the programs that work—and in the frustrations and failures that cry out for change.

Healthcare providers reflect on public policy issues from within a unique lived experience of these policies' effects and implications. Theologians realize that good theology cannot be removed from life experience. The people most deeply involved in life's struggles often have a privileged sense of their deeper meaning and importance.[23] It is important, therefore, that healthcare professionals reflect together prayerfully to understand their experience in its full social setting. What is God doing and inviting us to do—not simply as individuals, corporations, associations, or networks of associations, but as a nation and a people?[24]

Perhaps the most important answer to the question of how Catholic healthcare facilities and systems will shape public policy is through faith reflection on their identity and vocation. If, day to day, they together try to trace the Holy Spirit's movements, they will find themselves moved not only to a more sensitive healing presence to the individuals around them, but also to wise and more effective action in shaping the policies that determine the nation's health. It is vital to the U.S. healthcare system's future and to those who need its services that religiously committed healthcare professionals speaking from the foundations of their faith participate in the policy development process.

Footnotes
1. This chapter is a revision of an article published in *Hospital Progress* in May 1984.
2. John E. Curley, Jr., president, The Catholic Health Association, responded to this challenge in the article "Stewardship: Service, Management, Advocacy," *Hospital Progress*, November 1983, pp. 32-35, 51. He observed that if this largest single segment of the healthcare delivery system in American does not "get its act together," then "the entire voluntary healthcare industry [sic] may be lost.... Through our presence, we have the opportunity, indeed the responsibility, to shape the values of a nation."
3. "Action on behalf of justice and participation in the transformation of the world fully appear to us as a constitutive dimension of the preaching of the Gospel, or, in other words, of the church's mission for the redemption of the human race and its liberation from every oppressive situation." Synod of Bishops, Second General Assembly, *Justice in the World*, Vatican Polygot Press, Vatican City, 1971, #6. The document is available through the U.S. Catholic Conference, Washington, DC.
4. See Peter Henriot's discussion of global poverty and the nuclear arms race as the social contexts of healthcare today in Chapter 1. The federal government's invitation to hospitals to participate in a national plan to handle casualties in the event of nuclear war is one evidence of the thrust of the suggestion.

5. This is well documented in a publication from the Sisters of Mercy Health Corporation concerning the care of the elderly. See Andrea G. Jensen, "Challenges for SMHC in Serving the Elderly," Sisters of Mercy Health Corporation, Detroit, February 1982.
6. The legislation is entitled Reform Act for the Provision of Healthcare for the Medically Indigent. It was passed in the early 1980s.
7. That this type of statement captures the tenor of their approach was confirmed when Michael Novak responded to an earlier version of this chapter in a letter to *Hospital Progress,* July-August 1984: He ended that letter with the following paragraph:
    "The problem all of us face is how best to serve the poor and the needy. There are so many of them. There are so many ways to fail them—by imprisoning them in dependency, for example, instead of empowering them to care for themselves in simple dignity and liberty of choice. Fr. Hug and his friends have no monopoly on compassion; and they are far from showing how their dreams will actually work in practice. I encourage him to keep dreaming, while keeping one eye on what works. Dreams alone do not help the poor." (p. 10)
8. There are some remarkable parallels between the first two models developed here and the two viewpoints on social values elborated by Donabedian Avedis, MD, *Aspects on Medical Care Administration: Specifying Requirements for Health Care,* Harvard University Press, Cambridge, MA, pp. 1-30. The models are not identical, however, under closer scrutiny. Although a careful analytic comparison might prove interesting, the most important difference for the purposes of this discussion is obvious. The models developed here are explicitly theological models calling for explicit theological reflection and response.
9. See Robert Benne, *The Ethic of Democratic Capitalism,* Fortress Press, Philadelphia, 1981. Mr. Novak's theology reflects a policy line coherent with the economics elaborated by some of his colleagues at the American Enterprise Institute. See Mancur Olson, ed., *A New Approach to the Economics of Health Care,* American Enterprise Institute for Public Policy Research, Washington, DC, 1982. See also the insightful review of it by Eli Ginzberg in *Hospital Progress,* October 1983, p. 101.
10. Michael Novak, *The Spirit of Democratic Capitalism,* Simon and Schuster, New York, 1982, p. 355.
11. For Novak's position, see his letter to the editor of *Hospital Progress,* July-August 1984, p. 8.
12. This understanding of Novak's position on health care as a human right was confirmed in private conversation with him. For further general background, see the treatment of socialism and utopianism in *The Spirit of Democratic Capitalism.*
13. See, for example, the interview with Edmund D. Pellegrino, MD, director of the Kennedy Institute, *Hospital Progress,* February 1983, p. 355.
14. *The Spirit of Democratic Capitalism,* pp. 84, 124ff., 344-349, 353-358. Novak has not to my knowledge addressed the issue of for-profit healthcare systems. However, it is clear that his thought tends in the general direction described here. See his article, "The Communitarian Individual," in *The Public Interest,* Summer 1982, pp. 3-20, especially p. 19.

15. They included John Howard Yoder and Charles K. Wilber of the University of Notre Dame; William J. Byron, SJ, President, The Catholic University of America; Philip S. Land, SJ, Center of Concern; Patricia Mische, Global Education Associates; and Mary Evelyn Jegen, SND, Pax Christi.
16. Mary Evelyn Jegen and Bruno V. Manno, eds., *The Earth is the Lord's; Essays on Stewardship*, Paulist Press, New York, 1978.
17. 1 Jn 4:7-12.
18. Thomas Aquinas, *Summa Theological* II-II, Q. 66, art. 2.
19. Contemporary Catholic social teaching now speaks of a "social mortgage" on all private property. See John Paul II's "Opening Address at the Puebla Conference," Puebla, Mexico, Jan. 28, 1979, in John Eagleson and Philip Scharper, eds., *Puebla and Beyond*, Orbis Books, Maryknoll, NY, 1979, p. 67. It is quoted in the U.S. Catholic bishops' economic pastoral, *Economic Justice for All: Pastoral Letter on Catholic Social Teaching and the U.S. Economy*, #115.

    Recent studies of Judeo-Christian origins raise an even sharper critique. In *You Shall Not Steal: Community and Property in the Biblical Tradition*, Orbis Books, Maryknoll, NY, 1985, Robert Gnuse writes: "Thus, the command (not to steal) may have slowed the growth of individual ownership rather than protected it. The command may have meant, 'Do not take communal property for your own individual ownership.' How ironic that modern society uses the commandment to defend the opposite course of action!

    The purpose of the command was to curb those who steal from society at large by amassing great wealth for such theft will ultimately break down that society. This explains the ire of the prophets who inveighed against the wealthy classes of Samaria and Jerusalem." (p. 7)

    In *Ownership: Early Christian Teaching*, Orbis Books, Maryknoll, NY, 1983, Charles Avila traces similar themes throughout the patristic era.
20. A recent report from an extensive project study carried out by over 100 well-known U.S. scientists indicates that as small a nuclear exchange as about 100 megatons would create a nuclear winter—a cloud in the atmosphere capable of stopping food production worldwide long enough to virtually ensure the extermination of the human species.
21. *Health and Health Care*, National Conference of Cathlic Bishops, *Origins*, Vol. 11, No. 25, Dec. 3, 1981, pp. 396-402.
22. "Bishops want and need the continuing concern of Catholic healthcare professionals and need feedback on these life issues. The issues are complex, and we need to share our best professional, theological, and pastoral thoughts. We cannot afford the luxury of acting independently of each other." See Bishop Malone's article "The Church as Steward: Our Healing Heritage," *Hospital Progress*, November 1983, p. 31.
23. For an interesting development of this notion, see Larry L. Rasmussen, "Community Reflection," in James E. Hug, ed., *Tracing the Spirit: Communities, Social Action, and Theological Reflection*, Paulist Press, New York, 1983, p. 260ff.
24. For an approach to this type of reflection and a process for carrying it on, see Chapter 4, "Capitalism and Christian Values: A Process for Discernment."

Reflection Questions

1. Examples are given of the theology of democratic capitalism, the theology of stewardship, and the theology in the U.S. bishops' pastoral letter *Health and Health Care*, and of their logical implications for policy decisions.
   - How do you evaluate the theology of democratic capitalism? What are its good points? What do you disagree with?
   - With the theology of stewardship?
   - With the theology of the pastoral letter *Health and Health Care*? And why?

2. This chapter suggests that those engaged in healthcare ministry must strive to heal the church's and the nation's social structures as well. It points to the links between religious belief and indicates that theological reflection is needed to reconcile the differences between our faith and our social policies.
   - How do you imagine God? How do you identify God's presence in your life?
   - Can you perceive a new face of God in the midst of and despite the present turmoil in the healthcare environment? Explain.
   - How would you describe your vision of the healing ministry?
   - Could this vision find expression in public policy? How?

3. What structures and processes can be put in place to bring together the faith reflection of all the people in your institution(s)?

Discerning
The Appropriate
Responses

Discerning God's presence and activity in our daily experience not only clarifies our identity as religiously based healthcare providers, it begins to identify the concrete directions into which we are being called. What is the future of religiously based healthcare in the United States? That should not be seen as a question about the institution's fate as that is determined by economic, political, sociological, and cultural forces beyond our control. In the midst of all those forces, it is primarily a question about the call to ministry from God to this generation of healthcare providers, and about their personal and institutional responses.

The chapters in Section III attempt to offer help in discovering the directions of God's invitation. Chapter 4 outlines a process to be used in discerning the signs of God in our experience. It points up the importance of diagnostic analysis and faith reflection carried on in a widely participative manner.

Chapter 5 argues that the key to discerning the ministry we are being called to is the option for the poor. Grounding its argument in the Christian scriptures, it responds clearly and incisively to the flood of questions that usually arise in any discussion of this topic. The result is extremely practical and certainly challenging.

Chapter 6 expands the usual understanding of diagnosis, pointing out its inadequacy in the complex interconnected reality that is the context of our lives. It also develops further the notion of holistic health that has been introduced in earlier chapters. Without expanding our grasp of the nature and demands of adequate diagnosis and holistic health, we will not be able to understand the illnesses we are confronted with or discern the ministry we are called to.

The final chapter of this section, Chapter 7, develops a social diagnosis of our contemporary reality and explores some of its implications for future healthcare ministry. It is one model of the type of reflective and probing we are all called to, and it raises some important questions for us to mull over.

· 4 ·

Capitalism and Christian Values:
A Process for Discernment[1]

James E. Hug, SJ

Let me begin by offering two images. The first is a composite drawn from different factual situations that merged in a daydream I had last week. Diablo is a nine-year-old who lives just down the street from my community in a poor section of Washington, DC. He comes over frequently to play, to get help with homework, or to breakdance and do flips on our living room floor. Mostly, he comes for attention and affection. One evening, in my daydream, he runs in screaming. His mother has just been stabbed before his eyes. We rush her to the nearest hospital—a Catholic hospital. She regains consciousness on the way and seems a little stronger. The hospital learns she has no insurance. We are put in a cab and sent across town to another hospital. Diablo's mother dies.

The second image is from a photograph given to me. It shows a cement-block storefront. Above the door and show window, under the eaves, bold letters proclaim: CHRIST IS OUR BUSINESS PARTNER. Smaller signs have been nailed to the pillars on the front porch: "Keep Out," "For Sale," "No Trespassing." The caption under the picture is "The Hard Reality of Monday Morning."

Tragedy and Dollars

These two images capture a tension confronting health-care institutions. Dramas of heart-rending tragedy walk through the door every day. Yet increasingly people in healthcare are being

51

forced to look at that suffering in terms of the shrinking dollar available for responding to it. Is the hard reality of Monday morning, 2000, destined to reveal that U.S. corporate institutions that were serious about taking Christ as a senior business partner and policy guide were forced to hang out "For Sale" signs? Are the poor destined to die in taxis searching for adequate healthcare?

I do not have answers for these questions. But I do want to encourage leaders in healthcare to continue struggling for ways to resolve them. Catholic institutions are key actors in that struggle—a struggle in which far more is at stake than we usually recognize.

As a theologian I have become interested in economic issues through the years as I have watched the religious and moral issues embodied in public policy decisions dealt with predominantly in terms of their economic dimensions. That should create tensions and problems for people of faith, because we do not believe that economic efficiency is the highest human value.

The Microcosm

The struggles facing Catholic healthcare institutions today present a distilled and clarified microcosm of the basic tensions between Christian values and the capitalism that Christians in every sector of our society live with. They are the very tensions the U.S. bishops tried to address in their pastoral letter on the economy. How the Catholic healthcare community deals with those tensions and to what degree it succeeds could be of great importance for the whole nation and its economy. It could provide an illuminating precedent or, to use theological terminology, an important sacramental moment revealing graced ways to respond institutionally and individually to our current context.

If they are to survive economically, can Catholic healthcare institutions afford to make a strong commitment to serving the poor? Can they afford unionized labor, just wages and benefits, and good working conditions and still remain cost competitive? On the other hand, can they oppose any of these things if they are to remain truly *Catholic* institutions? Can they afford extensive programs of spiritual care when no funding sources are available for them and revenues are drying up? Can they cut back on such programs without losing their identity? What does it profit them to stand up as a prophetic voice and then not survive to provide any healthcare? On the other hand, what does it profit them to gain the whole world—including "the dominant market share of the healthcare market"—and suffer the loss of their soul?

I have sketched these dilemmas to show why I find the current struggle facing Catholic healthcare institutions important for the U.S. Catholic church today. Not too many years ago, Catholic healthcare had the space and opportunity to begin developing an institutional identity embodying Catholic social vision and principles. As reflection on that identity was beginning to mature, healthcare was pulled out of its relatively protected economic environment and pushed into capitalism's market economy. The problems and stresses that have appeared provide a practical textbook case of the stresses inherent in the relationship between Christian social values and capitalism.

The Macrocosm

Much is at stake. Clearly the survival of Catholic healthcare institutions is in the balance. So, too, is the future direction of healthcare in the nation: Is the return to a two-tier system inevitable? Or, to transfer these issues from a sacramental microcosm to the macrocosmic context: Can corporations and other social institutions survive if they attempt to embody the principles of social justice? Are the principles of Catholic social teaching incompatible with contemporary capitalism? If so, how are we to respond? Must we perpetuate a two-tiered economy in which the poor in our cities and rural areas and the poor nations and peoples of the world remain enmeshed in dependence and life-threatening squalor?

These questions have been posed starkly to indicate how much is at stake. They could be softened to stimulate a creative probing for new possibilities. For example, under what conditions can Catholic healthcare institutions profit from the true values and disciplines of U.S. capitalism while deepening their Catholic identity? What changes are needed in economic, political, and healthcare systems if both equitable distribution of care and reasonable cost containment are to be achieved?[2]

The Strugglers

There is another important way in which Catholic healthcare represents a microcosm of our society. Not only do the struggles represent in classic form the internal tensions between Christian faith and capitalism, but so do the strugglers—Catholic healthcare providers themselves.

These people include members of sponsoring religious communities and dioceses, chief executive officers, members of boards of directors, physicians, nurses, technicians, aides, and people who peel millions of potatoes and mop miles of halls. They include members of organized labor and management personnel who distrust unions. There are the patients, too, the people who come from all parts of society—and who go through some of life's most intimate and frightening moments in healthcare institutions. This cross-section of society can bring a full range of experiences and perspectives to the emerging tensions between Christian faith and institutional life in a capitalist economy. At the same time, the group is small enough, organized enough, and trained enough in teamwork to be able to collaborate in developing creative Christian responses to the current situation. People in Catholic healthcare also profess that a sense of Christian mission and ministry lies at the heart of their work. That fact gives them a shared foundation to build on.

This, then, is my challenge to Catholic healthcare institutions and organizations: Physicians, heal yourselves. Healthcare community, heal yourself. Gather the great variety of resources within your community and find ways to bring them to bear, in the spirit of your Christian faith commitment, on the dilemmas raised by the economic and political squeeze you are experiencing. Those stresses and tensions are undermining the health of your institutions and of the whole healthcare system. Find ways to restore their health, and you will contribute as well to the Christian healing of our entire political economy, providing the needed sacramental moment.

Since the problems are representative of our general socioeconomic ills, it may help to approach them as illness, as disease challenging Christian healers. This approach could include the following elements: (1) experience of the disease, (2) diagnosis and history, (3) professional consultation, and (4) appropriate treatment.

1. Experience of the disease. This can be put simply: Enter into the pain. Human beings do not like pain. We consider those who do to be emotionally disturbed. We have many ways to deny pain or to drug it out of our consciousness.

Medical professionals, however, know the importance of pain. It is the body's way of revealing what is wrong, what is threatening its well-being. I have watched a medical supervisor order an injection to counteract a pain reliever, sending a friend of mine back into excruciating pain so that a clearer diagnosis might be possible.

It is just as necessary in the stresses the healthcare system and the national community are experiencing to avoid a quick fix, the drugging of our pain. Society must enter into pain, experience it, listen to it described in all its dimensions, and learn from it.

Where is the pain? How is the disease of the current situation experienced *throughout* the systems that constitute our healthcare institutions? Attending only to the red ink that is hemorrhaging in administrative offices would be dangerous. We must listen as well to the experience of nurses, physicians, support staff, workers who have been laid off, patients—and especially the poor. I say *especially* the poor because it is the pain of the poor that society most easily overlooks or ignores.[3] As the recent Vatican document on liberation theology reaffirmed so strongly, the suffering and the cries of the poor are one of the principal "signs of the times"—that is, one of the main sources of God's revelation for our times.[4] It is a sin of our society that we block it from our experience, refusing—or at least failing—to enter into it and own it. We are, on the whole, unwilling to take responsibility for its healing.

Because we are segregated from the poor—in our neighborhoods, in our jobs, in our social circles—we do not understand their frustration and anguish. Our compassion is not touched in ways that could change our lives. That is dangerous if we are serious about healing the social illness confronting us. Where we stand on issues such as these depends to a great extent on whom we have lunch with, work with, play with, and live with. Someone once observed that the trouble with President Nixon was that he never took out the garbage at night. A lot of things would change in a hurry if everyone in the upper echelons of healthcare institutions, businesses, and government spent a week every year living and working with those on the bottom.

We are part of an economic system that gives privileged attention to the wealthy and the middle class. We do not yet know if it is possible to give preferential concern to the poor and still survive in that system. The dilemmas are frightening; the situation, life threatening. Yet the roots of the conflict are deep in our Christian heritage. When we look at those roots, we come to considerations that fit into the next stage of the healing process: diagnosis and history.

2. Diagnosis and history. In speaking of diagnosis, an important fact is frequently overlooked. Any attempt to diagnose what is wrong presumes an underlying image of what is right. A sense of what constitutes good health and normal functioning guides the search for the defects in healthcare. However, two seemingly conflicting images of the healthy institutional life compete for our loyalties.[5] One image is *economic* health, which is presumed to involve tough cost-containment measures and pursuit of self-interest, using all possible factors of comparative advantage within legal limits. The other is *Christian* health, which encompasses the quality of life and justice revealed within the institution and in its relationship to the poor. Jesus identified his mission in the words of the prophet Isaiah: "The spirit of God has been given to me, for God has anointed me. God has sent me to bring the good news to the poor, to proclaim liberty to captives and to the blind new sight, to set the downtrodden free, to proclaim God's year of favor."[6] He identified with the poor and outcast of his society, while calling the wealthy and respectable back to the social justice concerns so central to the prophets' message. For those who feel themselves called to heal as Jesus healed, an institution's or community's health must be judged according to the quality of its love and its preferential concern of the poor and oppressed.

This does not mean that concern for economic efficiency is unimportant. It simply means that this concern must be integrated into a larger vision of health and life. Economic well-being should not be given overriding significance. It must not dominate our diagnosis of the situation facing Catholic healthcare providers and Christians in other economic sectors who are attempting to institutionalize their values within the framework of the U.S. economy.

The basis of good diagnosis is a thorough grasp of the facts. A primary concern of the 1984 Vatican document on liberation theology was that careful study of the facts is too often shortcircuited by the simplified application of ideological principles (or conventional rules of thumb) to complex socioeconomic situations. That does not occur only when Marxism makes inroads in Latin America. It happens in a different form in this country, and we need not look further than the daily newspaper to find out how.

Current U.S. economic ideologies have roots in Adam Smith's free-market capitalism. As with all ideologies, their principles and presuppositions are regarded by adherents as having the status of natural or scientific "laws" that must simply be accepted and obeyed. Michael Novak, for example, insists that we now know how to create wealth; we just should get on with it, following the laws of human economic interaction that Smith discovered. Others prefer the "economic laws" of such varied economists as John Kenneth Galbraith, Lester Thurow, Milton Friedman, or Michael Harrington. We all have our favorite economists telling us the way things *really* are.

That simple fact in itself should give us reason to pause, as the Vatican suggests, and take an honest look at the underlying values, assumptions, methods, and commitments that shape our assessments of socioeconomic reality and the policy proposals that stem from them. Unless that is done, the current stresses will worsen and healing will be a distant dream. It is a dangerous shortcut to assume that stiff market competition, complete government subsidization, or some middle-of-the-road regulatory compromise is the best medicine for the current disease.

Capitalism and Government's Role

Free-market capitalism and the pressure for market solutions to rising healthcare costs trace their ancestry in part to John Locke and his view of government's role. This is how Locke described the roots of human community in *The Second Treatise of Government:*

57

To understand political power right and derive it from its original, we must consider what state all people are naturally in, and that is a state of perfect freedom to order their actions and dispose of their possessions and persons as they think fit, within the bounds of the law of nature, without asking leave or depending upon the will of any others.[7]

For Locke, government is necessary only because corruption exists. Its role is to protect individual citizens' freedom and property. That will allow the natural harmony of creation to reemerge—the harmony that results from the individual exercise of personal freedom.

That vision of the human situation is the foundation of the free market system in economic matters. Individuals freely pursuing their interest, guided by the laws of nature, are seen to function according to a natural harmony, thereby ensuring the common good. The common good tends to be defined as the sum of individual goods. Those most successful are those most in harmony with the laws of nature and of God.

One of the worst embodiments of this understanding was the social Darwinism dominant at the turn of the century. Andrew Carnegie, for example, argued that wealth was a sign of God's providential choice:

The millionaire will be a trustee for the poor, entrusted for a season with a great part of the increased wealth of the community, but administering it for the community, far better than it could or would have done for itself.[8]

The understanding of social harmony, the common good, and the providential activity of God that have evolved in Catholic tradition are different. From Augustine and Thomas Aquinas through Jacques Maritain and the tradition of social encyclicals extending from Pope Leo XIII through Pope John Paul II, individual freedom has been valued within and in relationship to the community of the human family that brings it to life and supports its development. Government has the positive responsibility to support and further the good of that community. The common good is not simply the sum of individual goods or individual freedoms. It consists of all that serves to foster the climate and the institutional structures within which a spirit of wisdom, faith, love, and cooperation can work to meet the basic needs of all and influence the development of every individual. The common good can require sacrifice of individual resources or freedoms if necessary.[9]

A further point to be made here involves intentionality. It is not enough to serve the common good only by pursuing one's own individual goods even when "individual" is defined somewhat more expansively to include one's family or corporation. Neither the government nor the "invisible hand" can adequately protect and foster the common good, the sense of community, in a society in which all the individuals (personal and corporate) think only of their own self interest. Recent experience in the U.S. is showing that corporate lawyers can usually find ways to turn any community-minded legislation to the service of corporate interests, leaving the public to pick up the tab. A renewed national commitment on all citizens' part to conscious and deliberate service of the common good is needed to balance our already strong commitment to individual liberties and initiative. The U.S. bishops are right to highlight that in their recent pastoral on the U.S. economy.[10]

In pointing to these two different sets of notions regarding society, the common good, and the role of government, I am just scratching the surface of a large issue, which is not the only one that must be considered. Others include the role of scientific technology in healthcare; recent cultural, economic, and political history; the privatization of religious belief beginning in the Enlightenment, with its attendant distortion of the relationship of religion and politics; developments in Catholic doctrine and moral sensitivity since Vatican II; and newly emerging theologies of the economy. I cannot pursue these here, but further study of them can contribute valuable hints toward accurate diagnosis and effective treatment.

3. Professional Consultation. Professional consultation is an important part of healthcare, as it is in other areas. The more complex and interrelated a system, the more essential it is to gather as broad a range of experience, insight, and expertise as possible for dealing with its stresses. This is the great advantage in the widely participative process used by the U.S. bishops to develop major teaching documents such as the pastoral letters on peace and the

U.S. economy. Whatever particular process of consultation is used, a number of considerations should be followed.

- Since restoring a healthy Christian life is the primary concern, the consultation should be carried on in a prayerful context. An atmosphere of prayerful gratitude and peace opens people to each other, frees their intuition, and guides their reflection and evaluation. Prayer certainly does not replace careful research, scientific analysis, or open communication. It does make it possible, however, for faith to throw light on the facts and analysis and to provide the ultimate criterion of judgment and policy formulation.
- The process should include input from all who are involved, especially the poor and the powerless, for two fundamental reasons: (1) "hands-on" involvement illuminates certain aspects of the truth not easily learned in any other way, and (2) the Holy Spirit resides in all of us and speaks in and through all of us, not only through those in authority.
- All involved must be honest and self-critical. All must be willing to ask, in the presence of God and with others, what elements of self-interest, personal anxiety, blindness, or prejudice govern their openness, viewpoint, or judgments.
- The process should allow time for the creative imagination to "play" with all the contributions, to dream about new configurations, structures, procedures, directions, and policies.
- The values each participant raises should be protected as much as possible and integrated in a way that fosters loving community service in the spirit of Jesus.

4. Appropriate Treatment. Effective treatment is still to be discovered; no cure is yet known. The healer's most important task is to help release the body's own energies for restoration and growth. These suggestions have been intended to facilitate that. The final outcome—healing or death—will be the result of the processes and future decisions of the nation's Catholic healthcare institutions. These institutions have already begun some imaginative and important initiatives at the state level. Many are finding ways to network to cut costs and increase their institutional ability to work for justice. Through communications networks they may also find ways to share expensive diagnostic resources both locally and internationally.[11]

Many institutions are exploring creative program possibilities that can better embody Christian values and meet people's needs. Some are considering exciting programs designed to seek out the poor aggressively. If networks of major Catholic institutions responsible for a large percentage of a region's healthcare were to agree to identify themselves so wholeheartedly with the needs of the medically indigent that those facilities' survival were threatened, they would give a voice to the poor that could not be ignored in that region or in the nation. If the struggle of one of the Big Three automobile makers could not be ignored,[12] neither could that of one of the major healthcare providers. This would involve accepting suffering, as Christ did, for the sake of bringing good news to the poor, liberty to captives, and new sight to the blind.

Finally, some hospitals have developed successful experimental programs in cooperation with local parish communities. This is an extraordinarily promising direction to take. As mentioned earlier, centuries of emphasis on market competition and the pursuit of individual self-interest have eroded community values and commitment to the common good. Many people from all parts of the political spectrum are calling for the rebuilding of the mediating structures and communities that constitute a healthy nation's essential infrastructure.

In its parishes the Catholic church has a massive network of community structures that could play a major role in that rebuilding, but their potential is largely untapped. Healthcare institutions must communicate biblically based views of holistic healthcare to clergy and religious educators so that these views can become part of day-to-day gospel reflection at the parish level. In addition, they should develop programs for listening to parishes' needs and for developing cooperative strategies to meet them. As a stronger sense of community is thereby restored, healthcare institutions should be able to call on the parishes for loyal support. Having shown dedication to parish concerns and to the church's principles of social justice, they have grounds to ask for a similar concern and commitment in return. They have reason to hope for support in lobbying and healthcare programs.

The Road Ahead

Catholic healthcare has entered a rare period of testing and choice that has profound implications for Christians in all sectors of our economy. The road ahead is sure to be difficult and filled with puzzling challenges. Christian values and capitalism: Where do they conflict? Where do they converge? What compromises are necessary? What compromises are possible without a loss of Christian integrity?

Catholic healthcare can take up these challenges confident that the Spirit of God dwelling among us is the source of great creativity and power to heal individuals, institutions, and society at large. At the same time it must realize that it will have no effective power to heal if it or the Christian communities around it lack faith and are too caught up in individualistic competition that sets them against each other and wastes our society's energies and resources. Catholic healthcare must call forth the faith of our church communities in cooperation with its own efforts and in support of them.

Finally, Christian healers must enter the struggle to heal our society with the peace and the freedom to lay down their work in healthcare if and when it becomes clear that this work hinders or limits their deeper Christian mission. That peace and freedom are possible only if they, like Jesus, are committed above all else to God's call and mission to them individually and as a community and are ready, as Jesus was, even to leave those who want them and need them when it is time to move on.[13]

Footnotes
1. This is a revised version of an article published in *Health Progress,* January-February 1985.
2. See Leonard J. Weber, "Ethics Commission Access Report Urges Adequate Health Care for All," *Hospital Progress,* July-August, 1984, pp. 62-65.
3. For more on the issue of the "preferential option for the poor," see Chapter 5, "Service of the Poor: The Foundation of Judeo-Christian Christian Response."
4. Sacred Congregation for the Doctrine of the Faith, *Instruction on Certain Aspects of the "Theology of Liberation,"* Vatican Polyglot Press, Vatican City, 1984, I.1 ff. For more on the signs of the times and their importance for contemporary Christian Spirituality, see James E. Hug, SJ, and Rose Marie Scherschel, *Social Revelation: A Profound Challenge for Christian Spirituality,* Washington, DC, Center of Concern, 1988.

5. For a fuller discussion of this topic under the categories of "industry" and "ministry," see Chapter 2, "Catholic Healthcare: Competing and Complementary Models."

6. Lk 4:18-19.

7. John Locke, *Two Treatises of Government*, T.I. Cooke, ed., Hafner Press, New York, 1947, pp. 9, 123ff.

8. Andrew Carnegie, *The Gospel of Wealth and Other Timely Essays*, Ed C. Kirkland, ed., Harvard University Press, Cambridge, 1962.

9. Leonard Weber forcefully makes the same point in the article cited in footnote 2 (see pp. 63-64). The latest official Catholic statement on these themes is *Economic Justice for All: Pastoral Letter on Catholic Social Teaching and the U.S. Economy*, National Conference of Catholic Bishops, U.S. Catholic Conference, Washington, DC, 1986, ##28-126 passim.

10. *Economic Justice for All: Pastoral Letter on Catholic Social Teaching and the U.S. Economy*, ##95, 295-325.

11. See Chapter 10, "Generating a Truly *Catholic* Response in Difficult Times."

12. I refer here to the U.S. government bailout of Chrysler Corporation in 1980.

13. Mk 1:29-39.

Reflection Questions

1. This chapter claims that people of faith do not believe that economic efficiency is the highest value.
   - Is it apparent to outsiders that your institution is "about God's business?"
   - What would you identify as the highest values reflected in your institution's life and policies?
2. A dilemma is sketched highlighting the tension between Christian social values and capitalism in these questions:
   - Can Catholic healthcare institutions afford to make a strong commitment to serving the poor? Can they afford unionized labor, just wages and benefits, and good working conditions and still remain cost competitive? Can they afford extensive programs of spiritual care when no funding sources are available for them and revenues are drying up?
   - On the other hand, can they oppose any of these things if they are to remain truly *Catholic* institutions?
   - Are the principles of Catholic social teaching compatible with contemporary capitalism and with the ultimate survival of Catholic healthcare institution(s)?
   What do you think? Why?
3. Catholic healthcare providers themselves are experiencing the tension between faith and demands of generally accepted business practices. This chapter suggests that Catholic healthcare personnel are a trained group able to collaborate and thereby influence U.S. economic and political spheres.
   - What common values and goals are present among Catholic healthcare systems and institutions in your area that could serve as a foundation for such collaboration?
   - What organizations exist that could foster this networking? How might your institution(s) cooperate more effectively with them?
   - Could a dramatic stand similar to that of the auto makers mentioned be made?
4. Most people live in environments in which they associate with others like themselves. Decision makers must come into contact with patients and with the personnel of institutions, most especially those of marginal means.
   - In your personal or professional life, do you have contact

with people of different socioeconomic backgrounds than your own?

- How can individuals be encouraged to open themselves to the experience, perspective, and pain, especially of the less privileged of society?

5. Gathering a broad range of experiences is essential to any satisfactory analysis of the situation and appropriate response. Such a process should be prayerful, honest, and self-critical; allow for creative imagination; and include the values of all, especially the poor.

- What persons or groups in your institution(s) exhibit the leadership necessary to initiate such a process?
- What persons or groups could or should be invited to enter into such a process?

· 5 ·

Service of the Poor: The Foundation of Judeo-Christian Response[1]

Peter J. Henriot, SJ

The gospels are filled with calls to serve the poor. In his ministry of proclaiming the Reign of God, Jesus gives numerous examples of reaching out to the poor and oppressed, the needy and those living on society's margins. He challenges his followers to a similar response.

Three of the best-known parables of the gospels center around the service of the poor. All three play key roles in the U.S. bishops' pastoral, *Economic Justice for All: Pastoral Letter on Catholic Social Teaching and the U.S. Economy.* The parable of the Last Judgment[2] makes explicit the connection between serving those in need—the hungry, thirsty, stranger, naked, sick, imprisoned—and serving Jesus himself. "In so far as you did this to one of the least of these sisters and brothers of mine, you did it for me."[3] As the pastoral points out, what is remarkable here is Jesus' identification with the poor: "[T]o reject them is to reject God made manifest in history."[4]

In the account of the rich man and Lazarus,[5] Jesus teaches that failure to serve the poor person at one's door is grounds for exclusion from the Reign of God. The pastoral reminds us that Pope John Paul II has used this parable more than once—including here in the United States at Yankee Stadium in 1979—to warn the wealthy and the citizens of wealthy nations not to be blind to the poverty that exists all around us in the world.[6]

And with the story of the Good Samaritan, we hear the praise of the outcast who takes extraordinary measures to assist the neighbor in need.[7] The term used by Jesus, the "Good Samaritan"—a term that many Catholic healthcare institutions bear proudly today—would have been shocking to his listeners. It would have sounded to them much as the "good communist" would sound to many in the U.S. today. But Jesus' point remains clear: whether Jew or Samaritan, whether capitalist or communist, what counts is the quality of love and compassion with which we respond to our world.

Clearly there is something powerful and appealing in the gospel call to serve the poor. It is a call that the contemporary church has formulated in the language of "solidarity with the poor" and "the preferential option for the poor." In this chapter, I want to discuss what this service of the poor means in terms of spirituality and mission. In particular, I will explore the implications of this service for the ministry of healthcare in Catholic institutions today.

Emphasis on Ministry

The parable of the Last Judgment offers a good starting point for our reflections on the spirituality and mission involved in the service of the poor. Its message is quite clear: Jesus is met and the Reign of God is realized through acts of service to those in need.

The *spirituality* consists in a drawing close to the person of Jesus as found in the person of the poor. The poor woman or man is a sacrament of God: a visible, tangible presence of God, a revelation of the Almighty in characteristics of weakness and vulnerability. Our faith and prayer cannot but be affected by such contact with God.

The *mission* is the establishment of the Reign of God, which is made possible because we receive it and are received into it as that inheritance prepared for us from the foundation of the world. Justice and peace, marks of the Reign of God, become realities when we meet the needs of the least.

For those engaged in the ministry of healthcare, the meaning of *spirituality* and *mission* as emphasized in the parable of the Last Judgment has special relevance. Service of the poor in and through this ministry has a primacy both in the tradition of Catholic healthcare institutions and in the contemporary expression of the church's task of evangelization.

It is important to reiterate that the activity of healthcare institutions associated with the Catholic Church should be characterized as "healthcare *ministry*" and not as "healthcare *industry*."[8] This is not to deny, of course, that Catholic healthcare institutions must be fiscally responsible, efficiently managed, and effectively planned for the future. It is a question of priorities, of primary guidelines, however, operating a healthcare institution based on an industrial model, i.e., primarily as a business, affects criteria for decision making and evaluation. This in turn sets a tone and creates an environment within which the caring activity takes place. By its very nature, "industry" emphasizes rationalization, bureaucratization, new technologies, and universally applicable regulations. "Ministry," on the contrary, is always personalized and human centered, even when concerned with institutional and structural issues, and it frequently demands a stance of self-sacrifice.

As modern society becomes more complex, the human service sector tends to replace "ministerial" models of activity with "industrial" models. For example, much of the contemporary policy discussion about response—at national, state, and local levels—to the needs of the poor uses language and imagery that reinforce the industrial model. "Safety nets" and "bottom lines" are not categories that are particularly compatible with the tone and direction of Christian ministry to those in need. One need only think of the incongruity of using these categories in any reflections on the parables of the Last Judgment, the rich man and Lazarus, and the Good Samaritan.

Thus, the conscious choice to emphasize ministry instead of industry in describing healthcare within religiously based institutions can help *transform* society at large. It is not unrealistic to suggest that if all U.S. healthcare institutions were primarily marked by personalism, community, stewardship, and respect for life and for rights, these same characteristics would flourish better in other institutions. In short societal health as well as personal health would be attended to. This is what I mean by speaking of the ministry's inherent power to transform society.

The Option for the Poor

Key to the conscious choice to emphasize ministry in healthcare is, I believe, the option for the poor. Service of the poor is integral in both the foundation and the orientation of a health-care institution that emphasizes ministry.

We must be clear that the "option" spoken of in the phrase "the preferential option for the poor" is not a passive reality but an active one. It does not refer to a variety of "options" available, among which we can pick and choose, much as we might pick and choose the "options" offered us in the purchase of a new automobile. Rather, the "option" is an action, a deliberate decision, a choice reflecting values as well as desires.

For many Catholic healthcare institutions, of course, the option for the poor is an active choice to maintain the tradition of their institutional or congregational founders. Many religious congregations were themselves founded expressly to serve the poor. To be about this ministry, the congregations subsequently established hospitals, orphanages, homes for the elderly, and other institutions.

In their renewal efforts of recent years, these religious congregations have frequently reiterated their dedication to serve the poor. This has been faithful to the call of the Second Vatican Council, which challenged religious congregations to "a continuous return to . . . the original inspiration behind a given community."[9] This accounts for the emphasis on the "charism" of the original founder or foundress and the "charism" specific to a particular congregation. As a result of this emphasis, the recent shaping of "mission" statements for Catholic healthcare institutions associated with these religious has highlighted congregations, special concern for service of the poor.

Pope John Paul II reiterated the church's commitment to service of the poor during his 1979 visit to the United States and in his travels in many Third World countries. During a speech quoted in the bishops' pastoral letter, *Health and Health Care,* the pope stated:

> Social thinking and social practice inspired by the Gospel must always be marked by a special sensitivity toward those who are most in distress, those who are extremely poor, those suffering from all the physical,

mental and moral ills that afflict humanity including hunger, neglect, unemployment and despair . . . . But neither will you recoil before the reforms—even profound ones—of attitudes and structures that may prove necessary in order to recreate over and over again the conditions needed by the disadvantaged if they are to have a fresh chance in the hard struggle of life.[10]

It is important to note that the pope emphasizes both *personal* sensitivity and *structural* reform in his remarks, an emphasis that, as we shall see, orients the option for the poor in very special ways.

It is one thing to express an option for the poor; it is something else to implement it. In moving toward implementation, probably more ink has been spilled (tears, too) and more words exchanged over the definition of the "poor" than over anything else. To whom do we refer when we speak of the poor as the focus of a special preference?

Who Are the Poor?

The poor are the economically disadvantaged, the materially deprived who as a result of their condition also suffer oppression, exploitation, and powerlessness. At least this is the definition that I believe is supported by scriptural evidence and theological reflection, by the declaration of church leaders and assemblies, and by the common understanding of people when they refer to the "poor."

It is true that we often do refer to persons who are not economically disadvantaged as being "poor." These may include people of some means who suffer loneliness or rejection; or young people who, although not experiencing material want, are deprived of love and understanding; or affluent persons who have drinking or drug problems. We frequently hear it said: "Are not these people *also* poor? Don't they deserve our ministry? Conversations like this are fruitless and frustrating if they conclude that "everyone" is in some way poor—materially, spiritually, psychologically, intellectually, emotionally, etc. It is more helpful, to restrict the definition of "poor" to the materially poor, limiting its application to those who in our society suffer economic hardships. Then we can rightly turn to others in our society with other needs and minister to them in their own right and not under the rubric of being poor. This is important if we are to understand that all people should be served but not all people are poor and thereby the focus of a "preferential option" for service.

Healthcare's Option for the Poor

I believe that clarifying the definition of "poor" has profound implications for healthcare institutions having a preferential option for the poor. First, it is clear what the option does not mean. It does not mean that we only serve the poor when we minister to them *directly.* So frequently discussion on service of the poor breaks down over this point. We really do not have to probe further contemporary society's complex character—and thus we provide ourselves with easy excuses—if we practice a simple reductionism that equates the option for the poor with full-time, full-resource, full-scale and immediate involvement with those who are economically disadvantaged. Such full commitment to direct service of the poor is usually impossible for most healthcare institutions and healthcare personnel. Faced with such a demand, these institutions and persons are most likely to throw up their hands in despair and continue business as usual. As I intend to make clear below, the service of the poor is more multifaceted than this and hence leaves far fewer grounds for excusing oneself from its demands.

Moreover, the preferential option does not imply any sort of "class hatred" or rejection of those who are not poor. It is true that this option does recognize the existence of classes. It does acknowledge that in our society nationally and globally there are significant distinctions between rich and poor, not only in terms of money but also in terms of power, education, opportunities. But dismissal or hatred of the nonpoor is by no means a demonstration of solidarity with the poor based on the Christian commandment of love. Neither is a romanticization of the poor, a sense that the poor are the repository of all goodness, all truth, all beauty, and all grace. No, original sin is fairly well distributed across class lines, and there are not grounds—theological or empirical—for the romantic notion that it is not to be found among the poor.

What the option for the poor *does* mean, I suggest, is a

threefold stance toward society that affects our judgments, advocacy, and evaluation. Each of these elements suggests consequences for the mission of healthcare institutions that seek to serve the poor.

Judgment

The option for the poor entails a perspective on society. Because of our desire to serve the poor, we try to look at what is occurring in society through the poor's eyes. Those of us who are not economically disadvantaged can never, of course, see the world around us as the poor see it. But we can make an effort to appreciate the perspective from which the poor view political and economic decisions, public and private policies, personal and institutional attitudes, and individual and corporate events. The perspective is described in Spanish as *desde los pobres,* where the preposition *desde* is roughly translated as "from," "from the side of," "on the part of," or "with the view of." I emphasize here not that the poor's perspective is the only true one, but that it is one that is frequently ignored, neglected, or relegated to a subordinate position when important judgments are made.

For healthcare institutions, such a perspective means, for example, sensitivity to how the poor react to the numerous regulations and voluminous paperwork connected with admissions, treatments, and payments. Or it means examining the "first impressions" given by medical staff, technicians, and other professionals to the poor who come for help. At a structural level, this effort to judge from the poor's perspective forces us to raise certain questions about national health insurance, for example, or about unionization efforts among house maintenance employees which might not be the questions raised by the nonpoor.

Advocacy

The option for the poor brings with it a bias in reaching decisions or settling disputes. In any point of controversy, there are always two (or more) sides with varying degrees of merit. One may enter such a controversy as an arbitrator or as an advocate. An arbitrator attempts a neutral stance, tries to listen equally to all sides, weigh all arguments, and judge which side appears, from the case's merits, to be more correct and just. An advocate, however, enters the dispute not neutral but biased, favoring one side over the other from the start.

In controversies involving the poor and the nonpoor, the preferential option means that the Christian is an advocate on the poor's side. Entering a dispute with a stance of such bias is justified because if the side of the nonpoor is in fact correct, it stands a very good chance to be heard more favorably and to win. This is true simply because in addition to the strength of its position it commands the strength of the power, influence, education, friends, professional assistance, lawyers, research, publicity, and much more upon which the nonpoor can draw. Indeed, even if its position is not correct, these very same strengths are available to the nonpoor but are almost completely lacking to the poor if they are left on their own. This means, in effect, that without the support of advocates the poor stand little chance of winning, no matter how correct their position may be.

How can healthcare institutions be advocates for the poor? As significant social actors on the local, regional, and national scenes, they have the potential to influence government or institutional policies. Rather than being merely neutral in matters affecting the poor—for example, Medicare or Medicaid payments or special programs for handicapped poor—Catholic healthcare institutions should be seen as clear advocates for the economically disadvantaged. Certainly the institutions should not be seen only as advocating in their own self-interest—even advocating for the poor out of their own self-interest—or only on the side of the more well-to-do and powerful.

Evaluation

The option for the poor provides a tool for evaluating decisions and policies. Following logically from the stances of judgment and advocacy is the evaluative question that must be asked of all we do: "What will happen to the poor as a result of this action?" This is certainly not the *only* question to be asked, and it may not be the *most important* question. But it is an *essential* question if we are to be about the service of the poor.

We might draw a parallel with the Environmental Protection Agency's (EPA's) requirement that before any major project is undertaken (e.g., new buildings, highway construction), an "environmental impact statement" must be prepared. This study must estimate the consequences such a project will have on the surrounding ecology. Similarly, the service of the poor demands a "poor impact statement," meaning that one factor by which we should weigh any project's worth or any decision's wisdom is its impact on the poor.

Healthcare institutions can serve the poor by raising this question when they evaluate current practices and future plans. For example, when current services are reviewed for renewal or termination (e.g., therapy centers, outpatient services), the institution should consider if the poor use these services. If a new clinic is to open, its location and hours should make it accessible to the poor. When expensive equipment is being considered for purchase, will such money take away from allocation of resources to the poor? Finally, how do employee policies affect the poor? With these and similar questions, a healthcare institution demonstrates that it is influenced by the option for the poor.

Practical Forms of Service

The threefold stance of judgment, advocacy and evaluation affects the perspective, bias, and questions that guide Catholic healthcare institutions in service of the poor. What does this mean in these institutions day-to-day ministry? What are the ways in which institutions can exercise their preferential option for the poor as articulated in their "mission" statements? Several ways in which a healthcare institution can serve the poor are as follows:

Avoiding Discrimination and Oppression

The first and most obvious way of serving the poor is for the institution to avoid practices that oppress the poor. This might be described as a *negative* solidarity with the poor: not doing things that are against the poor's interests and well-being. So many factors, structural and personal, impinge on the poor that it is important for us to be sensitive to whether we as individuals or as part of a corporate force are contributing negatively or positively to the poor's condition.

A healthcare institution that aims to serve the poor should obviously reject practices that discriminate against the poor. A blatant example of such practices is the advice given a few years ago by the director of the American Hospital Association's Division of Ambulatory Care regarding ways to discourage the poor from using hospital services. This is the practice of "demarketing," an effort to "cut demand from people considered relatively unprofitable in themselves or undesirable in terms of their impact on other valued segments of the market." Among steps suggested:

- Not listing the telephone number of the hospital emergency room.
- Providing little or no parking space for emergency patients.
- Segregating waiting rooms for paying and nonpaying patients and providing poor lighting and no food service in the nonpaying areas.
- Screening all nonurgent patients and sending poor ones to other providers.

The American Medical Association has formally disowned these recommendations.[11] But they represent an approach to delivery of healthcare services that has no place in any institution committed to serve the poor.

Certain economic practices of healthcare institutions—purchasing, for example—should be reviewed periodically to see if they oppress the poor. One thinks, for instance, of support or nonsupport of boycotts of the products of firms known for discriminatory hiring policies or of banks known for "red-lining" practices (refusing loans to poor applicants) or for socially questionable investment policies. Boycotts are controversial economic weapons, to be sure, but they can be effective ways to serve the poor by withdrawing support—and hence bringing pressures for changes—on institutions that oppress the poor. A positive approach to this same issue can be seen in "Project Equality" which encourages institutions to patronize businesses that have special programs to hire and train minorities.

Certainly the commitment to serve the poor also requires that healthcare institutions be just in their own hiring practices and in dealing with employee unions. Since it is especially the poor among minority groups who bear the brunt of discriminatory practices, discrimination on the basis of race or sex must clearly be avoided. Moreover, unions frequently are lowest paid employees only strength. Hence administrators should take great care to avoid an antiunion stance. Certainly management-labor issues are complex.[12] It is clear, however, that a Catholic healthcare institution that hires a fiercely antiunion consultant to foster negative attitudes toward collective bargaining among its employees not only goes against the principles of Catholic social teaching[13] but also demonstrates a lack of commitment to serve the poor.

Christian Attitudes Toward the Poor

The poor are served when a healthcare institution helps promote Christian attitudes toward the problem of poverty and toward persons caught in the trap of poverty. This is especially important when the nation's political mood is so insensitive to the plight of the economically disadvantaged. There is a "blame the victim" approach to much of the contemporary analysis of poverty and a "lower the expectations" approach to policy responses.[14] The poor are ridiculed (anecdotes about "welfare cheaters") or ignored (federal statistics redefined).

In such an antipoor milieu, Christian perspectives must be promoted at personal and institutional levels. To begin with, the charismatic vision of the religious congregation that founded the healthcare institution should be widely shared among all now in its employ. It should be inconceivable, for example, that persons connected with a Catholic hospital begun by religious sisters to serve the poor would display attitudes toward the poor at variance with the respectful and loving views of a St. Vincent de Paul, St. Louis de Merillac, St. Frances Cabrini, St. Elizabeth Seton, and Mother Catherine McCauley.

But even more must be done to promote truly Christian affection for the poor within Catholic healthcare institutions and to translate that affection into policies and practices. The scriptural and theological bases for the option for the poor must be explained to employees, making it clear that this is the guiding influence of the institutions' direction. Principles of Catholic teaching should be well known by all connected with the institutions.[15]

Promoting this attitude toward the poor requires a serious commitment to ongoing education and in-service training—as serious a commitment as is shown in the updating of medical skills and the learning of new technologies. The medical staff, boards, clients, and general public should also be helped to understand the attitude toward the poor that these institutions stand for and promote as a central element in their service to them.

Public Policy Advocacy

The poor are served by Catholic healthcare institutions when these institutions actively advocate for public policies to provide better care for the economically disadvantaged. The U.S. bishops' pastoral letter *Health and Health Care* made this clear when it urged Catholic institutions as follows:

> [They] should not hesitate . . . to initiate social action programs on behalf of their patients or potential patients and their families. Such programs will sometimes involve advocacy in the cause of justice for the underprivileged. This will include working for change in reimbursement methodologies which penalize and threaten the existence of hospitals which seek to serve the poor.[16]

As I mentioned earlier in this chapter, advocacy is a condition whereby we leave neutrality aside in a controversial area of public policy and take up a particular group's cause. It can certainly be expected that Catholic healthcare institutions would be advocates before our government in Washington, DC, for fair treatment of nonprofit health organizations, for safeguards against undue interference in administration, and for respect for life before and after birth. But a similar expectation flows from a commitment to solidarity with the poor, an expectation that these institutions would pressure the government to be sensitive to the poor's health needs. For example, this advocacy might take the form of legislative lobbying (within the constraints placed by the Internal Revenue Service on tax-exempt organizations) and of public education around social issues. It can focus on methods to contain and control costs and to encourage medical personnel to work in underserved inner-city and rural areas.

One way to ensure that advocacy is recognized as part of an institution's ministry is to take a look at the composition of its board of directors. Community representation from a wide background should be promoted. The board should be made up not only of representatives from business and professional fields, but also of representatives from ordinary citizens' groups, the poor, and employees of the institution. These people have important perspectives to offer regarding the stance of the facility. Although it is true that including representatives of the poor is not easy, it is important enough to be vigorously pursued. When the health-care institution is rooted in the community it serves, it is likely to be much more sensitive to the needs of the people around it—especially if they are poor—than when its direction is set by people outside the community.

On one of the issues that affects the poor, the bishops' pastoral letter *"Health and Health Care,"* was quite explicit. It called for the development of a national health insurance program. Without specifying what particular political approach to take, the letter nonetheless urged that "it is the responsibility of the federal government to establish a comprehensive healthcare system that will ensure a basic level of healthcare for all Americans."[17] Catholic healthcare institutions, in my opinion, serve the poor when they take seriously this challenge to advocate for programs to benefit the poor.

Outreach Programs

The poor are served by a healthcare institution through its ordinary and special outreach activities. By ordinary outreach, I mean simply the day-to-day practice of providing services to those in need, through emergency rooms, admissions, extended care, and so on. By special outreach, I refer to programs such as the establishment of clinics in poor neighborhoods and in rural areas where fewer healthcare facilities are currently available.

Most Catholic hospitals make it explicit policy that no one in serious need will be denied service for financial reasons. Urgent care to indigent patients is always offered, and no dying person is turned away at the door because she or he cannot produce evidence of ability to pay. Every day there are instances nationwide of service to the poor who come seeking medical assistance, service rendered *gratis* or with very little compensation. Indeed, many Catholic institutions today experience economic hardships because of the number of "charity" cases that they take care of.[18] This direct service of the poor is a distinctive and proud note of their ministry.

Another very serious problem that must be recognized regarding outreach to the poor is the fact that healthcare facilities are grossly maldistributed in this country. Inner-city neighborhoods and rural areas suffer a severe lack of services. This was one of the topics of particular concern in recent studies undertaken for the President's Commission for the Study of Ethical Problems in Medicine and Biomedical and Behavioral Research.[19] To meet the needs for more nonprofit and public community hospitals, Congress passed the Hill-Burton Act in 1946 to promote new construction through federal grants and the generation of matching state and local funds. Through 1974, the Hill-Burton program had spent more that $4 billion in federal funds on grants and loans for construction and modernization of medical facilities; it also generated an additional $10.4 billion in state and local matching funds for the same projects.

But despite its good intentions to encourage new efforts in poverty areas, the Hill-Burton program "was not successful in equalizing availability or quality of hospital services in urban and rural poverty areas."[20] Local community matching requirements could not be met, and many inner-city nonprofit facilities— including many aided through Hill-Burton funds—"have abandoned their service areas either by transferring their facilities to outlying suburban areas or by establishing satellite facilities in suburban areas which then drain resources away from the already resource-poor inner-city communities."[21]

If Catholic healthcare ministry is not to abandon the poor, it must seek creative ways to reach out to the poor, to where real need exists. Storefront clinics in poor neighborhoods, integral to a local Catholic hospital system, should, for example, be as prevalent as the freestanding emergency centers rapidly spreading into suburban malls. The Catholic parish system, in many instances very close to the people in need, should be used as a base for healthcare programs in conjunction with the ordinary institutional facilities.

Another significant instance of this outreach to the poor, especially important in our increasingly interdependent global community, is the outreach to the international scene. Mercy Health Services of Detroit has established an International Health Program through its subsidiary, Mercy Collaborative. The purpose of the program is to use the accumulated experience and expertise of the personnel of the Mercy system to assist the poor and underserved in developing countries. With a sensitivity to the uniqueness of other cultural situations, the program offers assistance in response to requests that come from governments, voluntary healthcare organizations, church groups, and so on. This outreach provides short-term consulting, developmental services, assessment and planning, and emergency services.[22]

Alternatives and the Poor

A final suggestion regarding service of the poor by Catholic healthcare institutions relates to the issue of alternatives.[23] The term *alternatives* is used in this context to refer to an approach to health issues that is at once traditional and future oriented. It represents a shift that is faithful to the charisms of early founders of Catholic institutions but is also open to the influence of more contemporary expressions of Christian values.

The alternatives approach is manifested in the "wellness" and "holistic health" movements. It is sensitive to the spiritual dimensions of healing and appreciates other healthcare professionals in society besides physicians. Prevention and education are emphasized, along with a community base for the healing process. Hospices and birthing centers are important in the alternative approach.

There has been considerable discussion about the alternatives approach in recent years, frequently arising from dissatisfaction with traditional approaches. Often the approach is looked upon as marginal to mainstream healthcare and is viewed with suspicion or even hostility. It has not always been seen as an important aspect of service of the poor. But I believe that there is a significant connection between the alternatives approach and the commitment to serve the poor today.

The ministry dimensions highlighted in the alternatives (e.g., emphasis on "high-touch" and not exclusively on "high-tech") can at times be more sensitive to the needs of the poor than some of the more mainstream approaches. The economically disadvantaged stand to gain much by an emphasis on prevention, education, community orientation, and integration of the spiritual, physical, psychological and social dimensions of healthcare.

Consequences

In concluding these reflections on the spirituality and mission involved in the service of the poor, I want to suggest some of the consequences of this type of service for the ministry of healthcare. These consequences are personal, professional, ecclesial, and societal.

At the *personal* level, service of the poor can be very satisfying, especially to the Christian who makes an explicit commitment to this service for religious motives. The most immediate satisfaction comes when we stop referring to the "poor" and begin talking about John and Mary, Jose and Maria. Poverty is "personalized," moving us beyond statistics to names and faces. For the many disappointing encounters in the service of the poor (and there are indeed many), there are many more gratifying ones wherein ministry comes alive in the mutual enrichment of the encounter.

There are also *professional* consequences, some quite unintended or unexpected. Special sensitivity to the poor affects the entire project of healthcare in an institution. Paradoxically, it can even lead to improved healthcare for the nonpoor, as an environment of love, concern, and respect for the human rights and dignity of all is promoted. In institutions where service of the poor is excluded or given only minimal attention, sensitive service of everyone else is jeopardized.

Ecclesial consequences may be more subtle, but they are nonetheless real. Service of the poor is a blessing for the church. Whenever the church in its leadership, membership, or institutions draws away from the poor, it suffers. History shows that periods of political division, doctrinal heresy, and spiritual shallowness have been marked by the church's identification with wealth and power and its distance from the poor and oppressed. Renewal movements have most frequently been accompanied by rediscovery of God in the "least" of our sisters and brothers. Catholic healthcare institutions renewed by a ministry in solidarity with the poor can be significant resources for renewing the entire church.

Finally, there are *societal* consequences. Catholic healthcare institutions serving the poor model a set of values greatly needed in our society at large. At a time of severe economic hardship in the United States and other industrial countries and of

81

disastrous economic conditions in the developing countries, the lot of the poor is very hard indeed. Public policy tends either to ignore or to exacerbate their situation. Therefore it is critical that influential U.S. institutions demonstrate a commitment to the poor grounded in the dignity and rights as persons. This is the truly transformative dimension of healthcare, since it heals not only persons but also society.

＊ ＊ ＊ ＊ ＊ ＊ ＊ ＊

These consequences are, in reality, signs of the Reign of God. When we encounter them, we encounter God active in history. In the service of the poor, spirituality and mission take concrete form. In the words of the economic pastoral:

> Christian communities that commit themselves to solidarity with those suffering and to confrontation with those attitudes and ways of acting which institutionalize injustice, will themselves experience the power and presence of Christ. They will embody in their lives the values of the new creation while they labor under the old.[24]

Footnotes

1. This chapter is a revision of Peter J. Henriot, SJ, "Service of the Poor: A Basis for Spirituality and Mission," in *Justice and Health Care*, Sr. Margaret John Kelly, ed., The Catholic Health Association of the United States, St. Louis, 1985.
2. Mt 25:31-46. See *Economic Justice for All: Pastoral Letter on Catholic Social Teaching and the U.S. Economy*, National Conference of Catholic Bishops, U.S. Catholic Conference, Washington, DC, 1986, #44.
3. Mt 25:40.
4. *Economic Justice for All: Pastoral Letter on Catholic Social Teaching and the U.S. Economy*, #44.
5. Lk 16:19-31.
6. *Economic Justice for All: Pastoral Letter on Catholic Social Teaching and the U.S. Economy*, #48.
7. Lk 10:25-37.
8. See the full discussion of this issue in Chapter 2, "Catholic Healthcare: Competing and Complementary Models."
9. Decree on Apostolic Renewal of Religious Life" *The Documents of Vatican II*, Walter M. Abbott, SJ, ed., Geoffrey Chapman, New York, 1966, p. 468.
10. *Health and Health Care*, National Conference of Catholic Bishops, *Origins*, Vol. 11, No. 25, Dec. 3, 1981, p. 400.

11. "Demarketing Speech Embroiled in Controversy," *Modern Healthcare,* January 1982, pp. 21-22. Cited by Ralph E. Peterson, "A Study of the Healing Church and Its Ministry: The Health Care Apostolate," an unpublished paper prepared by Lutheran Church in America, March 1, 1982.

12. For more on this difficult issue, see Chapters 8 and 9 of this volume. An even fuller discussion is available in *Issues in Labor-Management Dialogue: Church Perspectives,* Adam J. Maida, ed., The Catholic Health Association of the United States, St. Louis, 1982.

13. See, for example, Pope John Paul II, *Laborem Exercens, Origins,* vol. 11, no. 15, Sept. 24, 1981, #20, pp. 239-240.

14. See Charles Murray, *Losing Ground: American Social Policy 1950-1980,* Basic Books, New York, 1984.

15. A helpful introduction to Catholic social teaching is available in a handy book by Peter J. Henriot, Michael J. Schultheis, and Edward P. DeBerri, *Catholic Social Teaching: Our Best Kept Secret,* Center of Concern/Orbis Books, Maryknoll, NY, 1988.

16. *Health and Health Care,* National Conference of Catholic Bishops, in *Origins,* Vol. 11, No. 25 (Dec. 3, 1981) p. 401.

17. *Health and Health Care,* p. 401.

18. See, for example, the testimony of Edward J. Connors, President of Mercy Health Services, before the Subcommittee on Health of the U.S. House of Representatives on March 12, 1987. The testimony is available from Mercy Health Services.

19. For example, E. Richard Brown, "The Rationing of Hospital Care," an unpublished paper prepared for the President's Commission for the Study of Ethical Problems in Medicine and Biomedical and Behavioral Research, October 1981.

20. "The Rationing of Hospital Care," p. 13.

21. "The Rationing of Hospital Care," p. 14.

22. For more on this topic, see Chapter 10, "Generating a Truly *Catholic* Response in Difficult Times."

23. For more on this topic, see Chapter 1, "Building a Healthy Society: A Catholic Challenge of the Future."

24. *Economic Justice for All: Pastoral Letter on Catholic Social Teaching and the U.S. Economy,* #55.

Reflection Questions

1. This chapter suggests that spirituality means drawing close to Jesus, since God is revealed in the poor person.
   - Do you recognize the poor as a source of revelation, a sign of the times?
   - What is being revealed through them for us?

2. In day-to-day ministry, this chapter suggests an option for the poor can be exercised by avoiding discrimination and oppression, exhibiting a Christian attitude toward the poor, public policy advocacy, outreach programs, and alternative forms of service.
   - Identify several indirect, subtle methods of discrimination present in society, in healthcare establishments, in your institution(s).
   - What can be done in healthcare institutions in a positive way so that the poor feel welcome and comfortable in the environment?
   - How can operations be designed to extend healthcare services into the community more effectively? What role can you play in this process?
   - Does ongoing education and in-service training on the principles of Catholic social teaching exist in the institution(s) with which you are connected? If not, how might it be begun? If so, how might it be improved?
   - Is political advocacy on the poor's behalf recognized as part of your institution's ministry? What steps are being taken? What steps might be taken?
   - Do you believe all the people of the community should have a voice in the direction of the institutions serving them? How might that be done more effectively? Does your board of directors include people from a variety of social and economic strata in the community? What might be done to improve the situation?

3. The chapter cites hospices and birthing centers as specific examples of alternative delivery systems. Such alternatives are described as "high-touch," holistic, focused on wellness, and preventive.
   - Can you cite other alternative models that integrate the spiritual, physical, psychological, and social dimensions of

84

healthcare? What are they? How might they be implemented in your institution(s)?

4. There are personal, professional, ecclesial, and societal consequences of exercising an option for the poor.
   - What consequences do you identify as effects of serving the poor? Personal ones? Institutional? Ecclesial? Societal?
   - How does service of the poor improve the lives of the nonpoor?

·6·

Diagnosis: Good Healthcare in a Holistic Environment[1]

James E. Hug, SJ

Penetrating diagnosis is at the heart of effective healthcare. Without it, healthcare providers are reduced to the dangerous position of alleviating symptoms in the hope of restoring health.

A few years ago, a friend of mine was rushed to a major teaching hospital's emergency room with severe pain in his side and abdomen. One of the young physicians on duty judged the problem to be appendicitis; another was not so sure. Finally, one of them gave him pain medication to relieve his acute suffering. When I arrived, he was resting more comfortably. A short time later, however, a supervisor arrived quite alarmed and gave him a shot to counteract the pain medication. She explained that since they did not yet have an adequate diagnosis, it was dangerous to mask his symptoms. It would be better for his health in the long run for him to be in excruciating pain until they could be sure what the problem really was.

The problem, as they eventually discovered, was an aortal aneurism. If the supervisor had not acted decisively, demanding a full diagnosis, my friend might well be dead today. His pain was evidence of a serious problem in his cardiovascular system. Relieving the pain without attending properly to the systemic problem threatened not only his health but his life.

People relive that fundamental insight every day. Healthcare deals with the balances and imbalances of a person's *systems*.

No one who fails to think in terms of systems can provide good healthcare.

Systems

But what systems must be attended to for good healthcare? In recent years there has been growing recognition that although specialization has yielded rich rewards, in reality the cardiovascular system, the central nervous system, and all other body systems are intrinsically interconnected and interdependent. Good healthcare must attend to them all in a holistic fashion.

But is it enough for good healthcare to focus on these? Margaret runs a small clinic for refugees. Many children suffering from worms are brought to her. She has learned that the most effective treatment she offers is getting the families to dig latrines and insisting that everyone use them. These poor refugees from the countryside have no tradition of this type of hygiene. As a result, the children pick up the worms from playing in the dirt where others have relieved themselves. Margaret diagnosed the causes of the children's sickness in the people's social and cultural systems. Without addressing those systemic causes, there is little hope for adequate and effective healthcare.

And then there is the story of Ruben and his wife Marta. He was complaining of stomach pain; she, of sleeplessness. What does good healthcare prescribe? Maalox and Valium? What are the root, systemic causes of their symptoms? In the early 1980s they were living in a small village in the Salvadoran countryside. One day their teenage son was pulled from a school bus by the military and shot to death. He was to be a "lesson" to the other students. A year or so later, their village was bombed by the military as part of the counterinsurgency efforts. The people were forced to flee for their lives. Marta and Ruben have not seen one of their sons since that day. They believe he went to join the guerrillas. They relocated to another village, but two years later that village came under military attack. This time one of their daughters and her child were killed in an ambush as they fled. The rest of the family hid in a cave with little to eat for six months. It was during this time that Ruben's stomach pains became almost unbearable and Marta became unable to sleep. Their suffering forced them out of hiding and into a refugee camp in San Salvador to seek help. Two of their other children, who had been arrested for taking food and medicine to the campesinos in their home area, were now in prison. A day or two before I met them, another daughter had been abducted—probably by the feared Treasury Police—while on her way to visit her brother in prison.

What is the indicated healthcare for Marta and Ruben? Perhaps grief counseling is more appropriate than medicine. And advocacy, both in El Salvador and in the United States, for an end to the war may be the most appropriate healthcare of all for the situation.[2]

Good healthcare, then, requires understanding an ailment's systemic contexts—within the individual, in the family, and in sociological, economic, cultural, and political dimensions. It requires attempting to treat the causes as well as the symptoms, whether they are biological, cultural, sociological, economic, or political.

This certainly goes beyond the traditional understanding of healthcare providers responsibility—an understanding influenced by the dissection and categorization of the world the Enlightenment generated. And yet healthcare that is seriously and sincerely concerned to root out the causes of disease cannot simply medicate for worms without teaching about latrines. It cannot treat ulcers and sleeplessness without searching for ways to eliminate their causes. If it does, it must admit to treating only the symptoms and alleviating only the immediate pain. It cannot hope to heal effectively, and it runs the risk of aiding death-dealing forces by masking in the short run their destructive activity and power.

Closer to Home

Two of the stories just related come from El Salvador. What is happening closer to home? Is your census up for heart disease? For hypertension and ulcers? Are you seeing a rash of respiratory diseases and hyperallergic reactions? Do alcoholism, child abuse, and infant mortality seem unusually high? Are there more cases of indigent care than last year at this time? Frequently what all these have in common is a plant closing.[3]

If diseases like these result from a plant closing, a plant closing is a community health hazard that must be dealt with and, if possible, prevented. What are the root causes of these diseases?

What constitutes appropriate medical treatment? Advocacy for adequate healthcare for the poor is only a beginning of the treatment plan needed for dealing with disease-generating systems.

What about the cultural system of values that makes productivity so important to personal worth that it ties healthcare primarily to the workplace?[4] What sort of healthy economic system allows businesses to jettison workers with little notice or concern? They are in fact generally pushed to do so because of stiff market competition. And what of the social and political systems that seem unwilling to face the global changes affecting the environment?

Can good medical care, good healthcare, remain silent about these social illnesses that are the breeding ground for physical illnesses that absorb its resources and threaten its survival?

To put it another way, preventive medicine has social, political, economic, cultural, and religious dimensions as well as individual or personal ones. It must be focused institutionally and systemically as well as on the individual and the family. There are many more public health hazards than garbage and rats, and healthcare institutions must speak out against them. The census was up in Kiev in recent years for radiation victims. Can those who claim to offer good healthcare remain silent on issues of nuclear safety and toxic waste?

As we become more aware of the holistic inter-connectedness of life, those called by God to heal can no longer disclaim responsibility for dealing with the larger social issues or simply treat their effects or symptoms without failing in their mission and call. In recent years, the holistic health movement has focused needed attention on the psychological and personal-spiritual dimensions of good healthcare. It is time to expand our understanding of the human person and holistic health to include the essential social dimensions of spirituality and healthcare.[5]

A Salvadoran refugees said to me: "They (the military) bomb our land. They bomb our homes. They burn our crops and drive us off our land. They take us where we do not want to go—and they give us a little food and lecture us on how they are our friends." Sensitive healthcare workers will want to ask whether they play the role of the kind word and medication at the end of a distressingly similar social process in which displaced workers could say: "They milk us for all we can produce. They demand givebacks in salaries and benefits. They close the plants and lay us off with no warning. Then they give us a little unemployment compensation, some food stamps, a little 'charity care' at the hospital if we're lucky—and lecture us on not becoming dependent on society's generosity and welfare. And they expect us to recognize in them the gentle healing touch of Christ."

As people deeply engaged in healthcare pour their energies, commitment, and resources into healing ministries, they must reflect critically on whether their efforts are really good healthcare when the problems are diagnosed in light of the social systems that are their context. Do their interventions get to the sources of the problems and enable true human healing, true growth to human wholeness? Do they look beyond the physical, biological disorders, beyond the individual and the family groupings? Or do they unconsciously support society's disease-generating and death-dealing structures, institutions, and forces, allowing their dangers to remain hidden from recognition, perhaps even benefiting from their rewards? Do they, in other words, simply treat the biological symptoms of the disease among us?

The call to embody the love of God in healing care calls us to discerning care for social health and wholeness, for social justice and *shalom*.[6]

Growing Social Consciousness

What I have been describing as a contemporary challenge to good healthcare has analogous developments all around us. The stock market crash of Oct. 19, 1987, for example, revealed a great deal about the interconnectedness of the global financial system.

In the churches there has been some awareness of the importance and impact of social systems since the late 19th century, which saw the rise of the Social Gospel Movement in Protestantism and the beginning of the social encyclicals in Catholicism. Nonetheless, something new is happening. Between the first Catholic social encyclical by Pope Leo XIII, *On the Condition of Labor (Rerum Novarum)*, in 1891 and the second by Pope Pius XI, *On Reconstructing the Social Order (Quadragesimo Anno)*, 40 years passed. It was another 30 years to the next major social encyclical, *Christianity and Social Progress (Mater et Magistra)* by Pope John XXIII in 1961. Since then there has been a major document of Catholic social teaching every two or three years.[7] The church's social consciousness and concern are mushrooming rapidly. In the words of the Second Vatican Council:

> The People of God believes that it is led by the Spirit of the Lord, who fills the earth. Motivated by this faith, it labors to decipher authentic signs of God's presence and purpose in the happenings, needs, and desires in which this People has a part along with other people of our age. For faith throws a new light on everything, manifests God's design for the total human vocation, and thus directs the mind to solutions which are fully human.
>
> This Council, first of all, wishes to assess in this light those values which are most highly prized today, and to relate them to their divine source.[8]

God is active in the institutions and social movements of history, working to heal and redeem our world. A type of revelation is present in them that we are struggling to learn to interpret.[9] What is God doing and inviting us to do in the signs of our times?

The U.S. Catholic Church's efforts to answer that question are probably best revealed in the major pastoral letters it has produced in recent years. Through a process involving long study, wide consultation, and community discernment, the bishops have begun to evolve a theological interpretation of our social context that sheds important light on what God is doing and inviting us to. They certainly deserve serious reflective consideration by all who are concerned about the Christian mission of healing today.[10]

The Challenge Ahead

What began as a probing of the requirements of good diagnosis in healthcare has brought us to reflect on the social revelation and call of God in the signs of the times. To diagnose adequately and respond appropriately to the suffering person before us is the healthcare provider's participation in the Christian mission, a mission with fully interdependent and inseparable personal, interpersonal, and societal dimensions. We are just beginning to realize that God is calling us to an awareness of the sociological, historical, economic, political, and cultural context of individual suffering. All these dimensions are integral to it and shape it. They frequently play essential roles in its medical history, roles we ignore only at the cost of failing in our healing mission.

This is a new and somewhat daunting challenge, one that we must undertake together with the same pioneering spirit and courage that gave birth and life to healthcare ministry. A new age is opening before us.

Footnotes
1. This chapter argues that good healthcare requires healing attention to the social systems integrally related to human disease.
2. See also Unitarian Universalist Service Committee *Health as a Human Right in Nicaragua: The Impact of "Low-Intensity Conflict,"* Unitarian Universalist Service Committee, Boston, 1987.
3. See Barry Bluestone and Bennett Harrison *The Deindustrialization of America,* Basic Books New York, 1982, pp. 63 ff.
4. For more on this see Chapter 10, "Generating a Truly *Catholic* Response in Difficult Times."
5. For more on the social dimension of spirituality, see James E. Hug, SJ, and Rose Marie Scherschel, *Social Revelation,* Center of Concern, Washington, DC, 1987.
6. Shalom is the biblical term for the social wholeness and health whose sign is community peace and well-being.
7. For a good introduction to the tradition of Catholic social teaching, see Peter J. Henriot, Michael J. Schultheis, and Edward P. DeBerri, *Catholic Social Teaching: Our Best Kept Secret,* Center of Concern/Orbis Books, Maryknoll, NY, 1988. It contains an introduction to the tradition and an outline of major social teachings from Leo XIII through John Paul II, including important documents from Latin America, Africa, Asia, and North America.
8. Vatican Council II, *Pastoral Constitution on the Church in the Modern World,* #11.
9. For more on this theme, see James E. Hug, SJ, and Rose Marie Scherschel, *Social Revelation,* Center of Concern, Washington, DC, 1987.
10. Previous chapters have raised some of the themes from *Health and Health Care,* National Conference of Catholic Bishops, *Origins,* Vol. II, No. 25, Dec. 3, 1981. For some reflections on the implications of *Economic Justice for All: Pastoral Letter on Catholic Social Teaching and the U.S. Economy,* National Conference of Catholic Bishops, U.S. Catholic Conference, Washington, DC, 1986, for health-care see Chapter 11.

Reflection Questions

1. Healthcare providers are called to minister in a two-pronged way: in the short term they are called to attend to the symptoms; in the longer term, to address the deeper causes of the problems in all their dimensions.

   • How can healthcare systems' corporate strength be brought to bear on the socio-political, economic, and cultural ills of our day?

   • What persons or groups have enough distance to abstract from the immediate pain and illness to identify the underlying issues and causes behind them?

   • What is needed to help more healthcare providers develop these broader "diagnostic" skills?

2. A theology is not necessarily an intellectual construction elaborated in an ivory tower far from the life of ordinary people. It is simply a vision that confronts real events with the eyes of faith and attempts to discern the word that God wants to communicate through them.

   • How can people be encouraged to trust day-to-day experience as a source of revelation, a place from which future directions will be revealed?

   • How can healthcare corporations be encouraged to look beyond old certainties and securities, to examine possible sources of prejudice, and to explore new ways of channeling and providing the healing ministry needed by today's interdependent world?

   • What persons or groups could provide leadership during this time of transition?

·7·

The Socio-Medical History:
A Look at the Forces Shaping
the Contemporary Context[1]

Joe Holland

Our civilization is experiencing a profound social and religious transformation that has major consequences for the Catholic healthcare apostolate. This is the thesis I would like to explore in this chapter. In doing so, I will examine three problematics:

- The crisis of the social system
- The crisis of the religious order
- The impact of both on the Catholic healthcare apostolate

My intellectual work has been mainly with the crisis of industrial society and the Catholic Church's social role in the modern period. What I say here is an attempt to transfer insights from those wider fields to the more specific field of the Catholic healthcare apostolate.

The Crisis of the Social System

People will look back to the late 20th century as one of those extremely turbulent and transformative periods in human history, akin to the 16th century, which saw the birth of the modern world. We are now seeing what could be called the end of the modern world. Not that the world itself is going to end, but the period of cultural history that we call "the modern period" is now reaching its climax. Its energies are being exhausted, even in some very dangerous and destructive ways, as we see from the threat of nuclear war.

On the more positive side, the end of one age of cultural history marks the beginning of a new and different age. Our institutions must understand the nature of the transition. They must discern within the turbulence: What is creative? What is destructive? What is ambiguous? In other words, what forces should they resist, what forces should they purify (the ambiguous ones), and what forces accept?

I will look at the crisis of the late modern period from the viewpoint of industrial capitalism. More broadly speaking, both industrial communism and industrial capitalism are in crisis. I would argue, if I had more space, that they are in a converging crisis in which the worst features of both systems are converging into a single model. But here I will stay within the logic of industrial capitalism and see how it plays itself out in a crisis of the health-care system.

Three Stages of Industrial Capitalism

If we look historically at the evolution of industrial capitalism, we see the industrial revolution beginning toward the close of the 18th century. It takes strength from the middle of the 19th century on (the take-off period), particularly from about 1840 in this country. There appear to be three stages in its life cycle (Table 1).

TABLE 1: STAGES OF INDUSTRIAL CAPITALISM			
Stage	Laissez Faire	Social Welfare	National Security
19th Century	20th Century	Late 20th Century	
Capital Technology	Local Labor Intensive	National Capital-Labor Balance	Transnational Capital Intensive

1. *Laissez Faire.* The first stage has been described by social historians in the 19th century as the *laissez faire* stage of industrial capitalism. We hear a lot of rhetoric today about going back to the *laissez faire* model, but I do not think that that is what is happening. In the *laissez faire* stage, the government played a minimal role in the social economy. Its role was simply to let markets be free. It was a "negative government" in contrast with the mercantile systems, where the kingship controlled the whole economy politically, thereby inhibiting the creativity of free enterprise. Beating back the king's power to allow the capitalist entrepreneurial economy to emerge was a major step forward in human history.

Industrial capitalism in this period was marked predominantly by small, highly competitive family firms, using fairly rudimentary technology and high inputs of labor. It was a very creative and dynamic period. It was also socially ruthless. The Catholic Church took a negative attitude toward it, in part because of its ruthlessness toward labor. The great document of Catholic social protest against this period was *On the Condition of Labor (Rerum Novarum)*, the first modern social encyclical written by Pope Leo XIII in 1891.

2. *Social Welfare.* The period that shaped our life was what social historians came to call the stage of social welfare industrial capitalism. In this period we saw a new form emerge in which the state took explicit, although moderate, responsibility for the economy in the name of the common good. Particularly, we saw the creation of large state-sponsored or state-aided social services in the fields of education, general welfare, and health. We saw state support for collective bargaining and the rights of labor, unemployment compensation, social security and many more, none of which existed before.

This period was much more congenial to Catholic social thought. Although Catholicism had been hostile to *laissez faire* capitalism, it tried to cooperate with social welfare capitalism, especially through its schools, healthcare facilities, and charitable works.

The new stage was also paralleled by the rise of a new form of the business enterprise, the large, nationally oriented industrial corporation. It used higher inputs of technology compared with labor and was therefore, much more productive. It was able to corner larger segments of the market. If the first stage of

industrial capitalism could be described as the period of local, competitive capital and labor intensive technology, this second stage
could be described as the period of national, oligopolistic capital
and a capital-labor balance in technology.

3. *National Security.* Today, I would argue, we are coming
into a third and fundamentally distinct period that I would
describe as industrial capitalism's national security stage.

* * * * * * * * *

Each of these stages takes its name from the form of the
state. The state's function in the first period was to keep markets
free so that small family firms might compete. The state's function
in the second period was to balance and integrate the national
economy in favor of the large industrial corporations. It did this
through a working coalition of big business, big labor, and big
government. The state's function in the national security stage is
to streamline and discipline the nation to make it an aggressive
competitor in the world market system. It must do this because two
deep structural changes have occurred in the economy.

First and most obvious is that capital is now transnational. The world market system has matured. *Business Week* in
a 1971 editorial that it repeated in 1978, said that the predominant
fact of life of the 1970s is that the world market system has taken
on a life of its own, independent of national economies. This rise
of the world market system will have great consequences on the
healthcare system, particularly concerning state aid toward health.

What is the significance of this maturing world market
in the national security stage? It means that every government in
the world is forced to redesign the nation's internal life to make
itself an attractive investment climate for transnational capital.
Suppose you had $100 to invest in a bank. You go down Main Street
and find five banks, each offering a different interest rate.
Obviously, you would put your money in the bank having the
highest interest rate. In a certain sense, that is what is happening
worldwide as countries compete with each other to draw transnational capital to their boundaries, each trying to offer the highest
return on investment.

We know that businesses now examine carefully the cost

of Japanese labor versus American labor versus Brazilian labor versus Philippine labor, and so on. Labor costs around the world are running from as high as $25 an hour and more to less than $2 per day. If labor is too high in one place, capital will go where labor is cheaper. That is one of the main changes happening in the world economy.

The second big change is that the technology is increasingly capital intensive, and we are only beginning to feel the impact. We know of word processing in offices and the eventual use of robots in industrial production. We can speak of this as the cybernation of technology, the replacing of the human brain by the computer, much as the machine earlier replaced human muscle. One reason Japanese automobiles are cheaper and often better-produced is that robots are used in the manufacturing process. Robots can work 24 hours a day. They do not make mistakes. They do not require health plans. And they do not require pension plans. They do not form unions. They are considerably cheaper in the long run than human labor. The cybernation of the world economy threatens, unless deliberately steered by human values, to marginalize large sectors of the human family from any role in production.

Thus, two negative tendencies have occurred with the rise of the new stage. On one side, all nations are competing to see who can offer the cheapest labor. On the other side, all nations are pursuing policies of aggressive capital formation to invest in high technology, which may displace large sectors of labor from production and so broaden unemployment worldwide. According to the United Nation's International Labor Organization, as much as a third of the whole human family has been marginalized in a substantial way from production. They form a permanent under-class in the world economy.

Four Pressures on the State

In this new context are four pressures on any state, no matter what its ideology, from the maturing world market system that create the national security state.

1. First, governments are under pressure to produce conditions of *cheap labor* in order to draw capital to their boundaries or hold the capital they already have. This pressure is quite strong

because in many areas of the world labor is very inexpensive. Labor can be kept cheap in several ways. Generally this is accomplished by destroying working people's social and political power. One of the leading edges of this effort is the worldwide attack on the principle of free trade unions. We see this attack in both capitalist and communist countries.[2] By breaking working people's political and organizational power, it is easier to drive down wage rates.

Cheap labor can also be achieved by tolerating wide margins of unemployment. Working people as a result have less bargaining power. People are less willing to protest or go on strike if there are a thousand people waiting outside the gate to take their jobs. Today there seem to be deliberate social policies to maintain wide margins of unemployment.

Finally, it is also possible to achieve cheap labor by substituting high technology for human labor. There is an accelerating tendency in our country to use computers and machines instead of people. For a while the displacement of human labor from the industrial sector was absorbed by the growing service sector, but efforts now exist to curtail the service sector as well because of pressure.

2. The second pressure generating the national security state is *the pressure to maintain low taxes.* A political jurisdiction must offer low corporate taxes or low taxes for investors to attract capital to its area or hold capital there. Why? Because the higher the taxes on the investment, the lower the return. If Brazil is offering tax incentives for investing there and the United States is charging a 25 percent tax on investment, the U.S. is going to bite into the profit margin and Brazil is going to subsidize it. All nations are being forced to compete for investors based on attractive tax packages.

If employers are trying to reduce labor costs and if tax incentives to corporate investors are reducing the funds available for the social welfare sector, this presents a triple problem for the healthcare system. First, ordinary people's direct purchasing power is declining. They will not be able to purchase as many healthcare services. Second, employers will be looking for ways to curtail their own healthcare costs through competitive bidding. Finally, the state is likely to dismantle large sectors of its social welfare operation, especially in the healthcare sphere.

3. The third pressure felt by governments in the national

security stage is the pressure to *increase military spending*. Why are they pressured in that direction? The maturing of the world market system has undermined American economic hegemony and, therefore, American political and military hegemony over the world market system.

What was called once the *Pax Americana*—the stable framework of state relationships that was imposed after World War II by American global power—is in shambles. The world economy is now disorganized and volatile. Wars can spring up at any place at any moment because there is no imperial power presiding over the world, as there was under the Roman Empire, under the British Empire, after World War II under the American Empire. Yet all nations are now living in an interdependent world economy and have vital stakes in certain resources and markets beyond their boundaries. They must be able to guarantee investors that they can defend their role in the world market system militarily or else they will not provide an attractive investment climate. Indeed, their own national economic security will be in jeopardy. For example, the lifeblood of the industrial system, petroleum, is a great military concern. Where is petroleum? Especially in the Middle East and in the Caribbean Basin (reaching down into Central America). Where are the two military "hot spots" in the world today? The Middle East and the Caribbean Basin.

The expansion of military spending is thus a function of a volatile, unregulated, and interdependent world economy. If taxes are reduced to draw corporate investors at the same time there are pressures to increase military spending, there will be further severe pressures to reduce government spending for social services such as healthcare.

4. The fourth factor creating the national security state is the pressure on governments to guarantee what investors call *political stability*. Governments must control their political environments to make them attractive investment climates.

For example, if wide margins of unemployment are tolerated, the middle class is driven into downward mobility, policies of ecological recklessness are pursued, the social welfare state is dismantled, and aggressive military policies are advanced, there will be protest. That protest is likely to disrupt the economy. There can be riots and strikes. At the extreme there could be a revolution, a civil war. Investors do not like to invest in a climate where there might be riots or a revolution. Increasingly, transnational corporations are looking for stable countries in which to invest. They used to look in Third World dictatorships or even in communist governments like Poland. But the Third World and communist countries are increasingly volatile. There is great pressure to tighten control over the political systems.[3] The police state is not uncommon.

These four pressures—the pressure for cheap labor, low taxes, increased military spending, and "political stability"—are creating severe strains on the healthcare system. People are having a harder time affording it. Employers are streamlining healthcare plans to increase their competitiveness in the world market system. Governments are trying to curtail their subsidies to the healthcare system to make their jurisdictions more attractive to investors. The expansion of military spending has eaten into the limited resources available for the healthcare system. All these facets comprise the crisis of the social system.

The Crisis of the Religious Order

The Catholic healthcare system was founded principally by religious orders of women. Most of these orders were born either out of the French Revolution or the Industrial Revolution to minister to European peasants displaced by the rise of industrial society. We have now gone through a cycle in which those orders, unless major changes occur, are coming to the end of their life cycle. We are experiencing the very serious decline of the modern apostolic orders that emerged in the 16th century and through the industrial period. The crisis is particularly acute among orders of women in social ministries.

It is important to recall the history of the religious order so that we will not be too frightened by this death phase that one form of the religious order is entering. We must understand that the religious order can also be regenerated.

There was no religious order during the first three centuries of Christian history from Pentecost until the Constantinian marriage of the Catholic Church with the Roman Empire. Religious orders were not founded by Jesus and did not come directly from an apostolic foundation. There were no religious orders in the first three centuries of Christianity because all Christians formed what we mean today by a religious order. All Christians were "not of the world." All Christians belonged to a counterculture that stood in a hostile tension with the main value system of the world. It was only when, under Constantine, Christianity became officially recognized as the religion of the Roman Empire that it was assimilated into the logic of Western culture and ceased to be a counterculture.

I believe that the Spirit of God led Christianity into that marriage with Western culture. It could be spoken of as a covenant with Greco-Roman culture. It was positive and accomplished much. But it also had a negative underside. During the period of its marriage with the social structures of the West, Christianity was compromised and could not witness to the fullness of the Gospel of Jesus Christ. Therefore, it was necessary that some remnant hold visible the image of Christianity as a counterculture and "leave the world." This fell to the newly created religious orders, which then went through several historical forms.

History of the Religious Order

The first historical form was lived out by the *hermits*. They left the Roman Empire with its compromised Christianity and went into the desert to witness to the crucifixion. They quickly found that they were not alone in the desert. People left the city to be with them and to be guided by their spiritual wisdom. They had to feed and care for these people and put a roof over their heads. Thus emerged what came to be known as the common life or *monasticism*, the second historical form of religious order. The monastic form of religious life reigned the late years of the Roman Empire and through the early period of feudalism.

By the 13th century, a new postfeudal society was emerging, not completely under church control. This involved the rise of the commercial cities that traded with the East and, eventually, with the New World. A new social experience grew up around those cities. Universities were part of that newness, and the modern healthcare system grew out of them.

The monasteries were isolated from the cities. The city would not come to the monastery and so the monastery did not minister to the city. A new form of the religious order was therefore needed. This new form was called *mendicant,* typified by the Franciscans and the Dominicans. They lived in monasteries, but they left the monastery to bring the Gospel to the city. When their energies waned, they returned to the monastery. The city was a foreign place to which the mendicants went for ministry, but they drew their life from the cloister.

The mendicant's logic was stretched to the breaking point in the 16th century by the creation of the Society of Jesus, the Jesuits. The 17th through 19th centuries saw the appearance of countless social welfare orders, especially of women. The mendicant principle was abandoned, and the religious order planted within the world itself. These apostolic orders anticipated the social welfare state: they built schools; they built hospitals; they ran charitable programs for orphans and widows.[4]

Contemporary Religious Life

Today we are on the verge of a powerful transformation in the meaning of the religious order. We are entering a period in which Christians must once again form a counterculture. This must occur not out of hatred of the world on some ideological ground, but out of a loving concern for a society heading on a course of destruction. To save the world, we must mount a massive criticism of the way it is going.

As Pope John Paul II has repeated in his writings, we are developing the most sophisticated technological and scientific society the world has ever known. Instead of saving us, however, this technological and scientific society is now poised against us like a weapon. We are slowly polluting the ecology. Even worse, we are threatening the world with nuclear holocaust. In the interim, we are marginalizing the poor and turning against labor. Thus, the pope and much if not all of the church believe that Western civilization is heading toward destruction. Because we love the world so much, our task is to turn Western civilization in a more loving and creative direction. But to do that we must set ourselves outside the dominant culture.

We needed religious orders as a separate way of life when Christianity was part of the dominant culture. That led to a theory of "two states in life." "Religious" were those people charged with religion. The rest of us were the "laity," who dabbled in it. The relationship between religious and laity was similar to that between physicians and their patients. The theory of the two states in life, however, is now beginning to break down. Attention is being focused primarily on the one foundational state in life, the baptismal vocation. All Christians are called to become part of a counterculture that tries to steer the civilization in a different direction. We no longer need a remnant that distinguishes itself from the main lines of a Christianity compromised with the world, because Christianity is less and less able to live with the compromises being demanded. It is increasingly distancing itself from the dominant culture.

A New, Pluralistic, Lay Model

Does that mean that the religious order will simply disappear? Probably not, but it will redefine itself. Rather than considering itself part of a separate and distinct state in life, the new religious order will become a leaven in the midst of the wider church, stimulating and serving the entire church's prophetic energies.

This new form of the religious order will be explicitly *lay in character*. It will not distinguish itself qualitatively from other Christians but, rather, in the intensity with which it lives the Christian life. For example, a pioneering model of the new form of the religious order is *Opus Dei*. In a short period it has grown to more than 79,000 members around the world and plays a major role in the life of the church. *Opus Dei* is building very rapidly, recruiting new members while the traditional religious orders are declining. Why? Because it is building on the lay principle. Another example is Maryknoll. Maryknoll priests, brothers, and sisters are getting few vocations. They are ordaining a handful of priests a year, professing a few sisters and brothers. In the meantime they have started an experiment called the Lay Missionary Program. They have been flooded with applications. They are now sending hundreds of people into the field as lay missionaries.

Further, the new lay model is pluralistic. It includes men and women, singles and married together in a common community. It also includes people who are willing to make short-term, medium-term, and lifelong commitments in a pluralistic community of many styles.

104

Old religious orders may readapt to this new model. For example, many Dominicans adapted to the modern activist order and ceased to be mendicants. Benedictines are teaching in schools, although they really had nothing to do with schools in the time of Benedict and the Benedictine monasteries.

This is the crisis of the religious order. Many Catholic healthcare systems were founded under the old model of the religious order. Now that model is fading. It can no longer continue its former work. How is the Catholic healthcare apostolate to adjust to that reality?

The Impact on the Catholic Health Apostolate

Our third problematic concerns the future of the Catholic health apostolate in the light of the first two problematics: the crisis of industrial society and the crisis of the religious order.

A few years ago, someone working in healthcare said to me, "We talk about helping the Catholic system survive in a very dangerous climate." He thought we should instead be talking about "pioneering an entirely different system whose dynamic implications would spread across the whole healthcare system and across the whole world." He said, "We should not simply be talking about surviving, but rather of imaginatively unleashing creative energies that will change the very nature of both the Catholic and secular healthcare systems." I, too, believe that this is the prophetic vocation of Catholic healthcare.

Four Future Scenarios

Clement Bezold, an analyst linked to the World Futurist Society, has suggested four future scenarios for the health system.

1. The first scenario is an optimistic one: *continued growth and expansion.* This would be typified by the writings of futurologists like Herman Kahn. It is a continuous growth model. If we have a little disorientation in the system now, it is only transitory. We will overcome it quickly by doing the same things we have always done. We will have more and bigger and better hospitals, more health services, and so on. Most of us, however, feel that the future is more complex than this scenario suggests.

2. The second scenario is the flip side of optimism: a scenario of *decline and stagnation,* as sketched by the *Global 2000*

Report. The existing healthcare system, continuing under present assumptions, will become more crisis ridden and slowly decrease in its ability to serve people. It will stagnate into a slow but steady decline. This seems too bleak a scenario to lead us into the future.

3. The third scenario might apply more to the British healthcare system, where the state has played a major role, and, closer to home, the Canadian healthcare system. This is the scenario of *discipline.* It is clear that the present healthcare system has certain limits. It is becoming more expensive and must be curtailed in light of the national security context. The state itself will impose the discipline by drawing clear limits for the health-care system and will, in a rigid and bureaucratic fashion, distribute that limited healthcare resource to the whole population. This is George Orwell's model of the healthcare system in *1984*. It reflects socialist nations' tendency to respond to the crisis by stronger bureaucratic discipline, whereas stagnation and decline would be the tendency in capitalist countries.

4. The fourth scenario is the *transformational model.* This does not simply ask how we can subsidize the participation of the poor in the existing healthcare system. Rather, it explores the possibilities for a different healthcare system that will empower all people and transform both health and the whole society. It is this scenario that I would like to propose.

Building on the analysis of the crisis of the social system and the crisis of the religious order, what are some of the strategic implications for the Catholic healthcare apostolate? Following are my suggestions in the form of several transformational principles.

1. *The religious vision of the Catholic healthcare system in the future will be carried by the laity.* That does not mean that we will not have women religious in it, but we will not be able to count on a large number or a centrally positioned body of people like the religious in the past.

Compared with bishops, popes, and parish priests who have often been terrified of lay people, the sisters have been wonderful in reaching out to embrace laity. But the sisters have looked to lay people for what might be called "supplementary competence." The sisters established the religious vision and then attracted lay people to help with the medical, administrative, and financial work. The difference in the future will be the reliance on the laity for the religious vision as well. There will not be any new vision unless it comes from religious energies. The only realities powerful enough to challenge a civilization's direction, or the misdirection, are religious energies. And religious energies in the future will come increasingly from the laity.

Arnold Toynbee argues that at the foundation of every civilization is a religious vision. Therefore, the unleashing or the transformation of the religious vision at the foundation of the West is the first step toward transforming the civilization and, within it, the healthcare apostolate. Therefore, in the emerging age of the laity, religious communities should stress the religious formation of their lay associates and staff.

2. *The form of ownership and management of the Catholic health-care system should be increasingly cooperative.* I understand the cooperative movement as something that is neither the free market model nor the state-socialist model. It is something in between, rooted in the community of people who make up a given institution. A cooperative form of organization set up in the style of participatory democracy links those who have the gift of specialized skills with the general employees and with the broad consumer public that it serves in a common community of participation and decision making. The model offered by cooperatives can reroot the institution in the community.

I recommend a film produced by the British Broadcasting Corporation called *The Mondragon Experiment.* It tells the story of a group of Basque people in the north of Spain. Beginning under the inspiration of Catholic social principles, they built (and are still building) a powerful network of industrial cooperatives. In addition, an infrastructure of educational and healthcare institutions serves it. They have their own university and their own research center. They even use and design robots. No one is ever laid off. The system is built in service of the community. *The Mondragon Experiment* suggests that it may be feasible to pursue a model of ownership and organization based on cooperatives in a way that is more viable than either the state-centered or the market-centered models that dominate the crisis of late industrial civilization. I suggest that before the recent crisis, all institutions were implicitly rooted in a cooperative framework and that the free market and the state were only a thin veneer above them. But the roots in community have been dissolved more and more, until a rootless bureaucratic model dominates both private and public enterprise. Both forms now repress community and dissolve people's participation in it.

The pursuit of a cooperative communitarian model in the formal organization of Catholic healthcare systems might be very beneficial. It deserves serious consideration.

3. *The shift in the dominant scientific paradigm of the whole society, including medical science.* Insofar as medicine has been the leading edge of Western science, the shift is more acutely felt there. The definition of science that we have known in the modern world began in the 16th-century Enlightenment. Other definitions of science existed before then, and we are coming to a different definition of science now. I suggest that some contrasts exist between the Enlightenment model of science within the field of medicine and what might be a post-Enlightenment or postmodern model of science in the period we are entering.

First, the reigning model of science is *reactive*. If a problem arises, science tries to address it with drugs, radiation, or surgery. Although these are useful tools, we must supplement them with *prevention*. The alternative model is preventive. If our society hopes to reduce healthcare costs, it must realize that it is cheaper to prevent problems than to react to them. We know, for example, that many medical problems are environmentally induced. They could be stopped at their source. The dimension of prevention must be fundamental in a postmodern medical system.

Second, the existing scientific model of medicine is increasingly *specialized*. We break things up into parts and refine them. It is a mechanistic model. Health is not simply the sum of multiple specializations, however. Health is also a function of the whole—of the material whole of the body and also of its spiritual dimension. Modern scientific medicine is increasingly specialized. Postmodern scientific medicine must be increasingly *holistic*. That does not mean that we should bypass the great insights gained by specialization. Rather, we should try to understand how specialization functions within the complex concert of the whole.

How might the Catholic healthcare system marry faith and science in a holistic synthesis?

Third. the existing healthcare system is increasingly *technocratic*. It may be well-intentioned about having everybody participate. It may have an open-door management policy. But it is nonetheless increasingly technocratic. Those who hold the most sophisticated skills control the situation. Is the reverse possible— that those who possess the most sophisticated skills could help spread these skills across the whole community? We get a better sense of this by looking at what is happening in the parish. In the old days the parish priest was a monarch who controlled every-thing. Now in some parishes, a priest may have 100 lay ministers. They give out communion. They minister to the sick. They are in social welfare. Lay ministers are everywhere. In turn, the theolog-ical institutes are flooded with lay ministers wanting training. The religious skills once concentrated only in religious professionals are now being diffused throughout the whole community again. This is the way it was in the primitive church.

The parish priest can take one of two attitudes in this context. He can say, "They are undermining my authority here and I am losing my role." Or, he can realize that he is becoming a minibishop. He has a community of ministry to facilitate and organize. He can take a more relaxed approach toward life and enjoy it. Ministry is no longer just his burden. It is the community's responsibility.

The same shift is beginning in the healthcare field. From the birth of the modern Enlightenment, scientific skills in health-care were progressively concentrated in the physicians. This unleased tremendous scientific advances, for which we should be grateful. Nonetheless, the process also uprooted the healthcare system from the community. Now we are beginning to say, "Build on those tremendous scientific gains in healthcare, but diffuse those health skills through paraprofessionals and other forms of healthcare ministry back into the community again." Physicians will increasingly feel themselves the victims of a growing medical "anticlericalism" until they accept this shift. Therefore the future system would be *participatory*, not technocratic.

Fourth, the reigning system is presided over by a classic philosophy of *management*. We will certainly need managers in the future, but a different kind. Management, as it has been con-structed by liberal theory, has as its purpose holding parts in tension together and presiding over them without worrying about strategic direction. The importance of strategic planning is again becoming clear, however. Strategic planning must be creative, cooperative, and comprehensive. The vision that informs it must flow from an imaginative artistic *creativity.*

Fifth, the present scientific health system is *hospital focused.* Hospitals will remain vital, but as servants of a broader process. The future scientific health system will be increasingly *community focused.* What might this mean for the Catholic health-care apostolate? One possibility involves the relationship between the hospitals and parishes. Imagine a healthcare system with a two-way feeding process between parish and hospital. In an informal way, that is beginning to happen in some areas. A courageous woman founded a health clinic for the poor in downtown Washington, DC. She enlisted informal support from her home parish and from a local hospital. What if both institutions—the hospital and perhaps a cluster of parishes—were to take seriously the sponsorship of a clinic like this? The energies and finances that would be mobilized could be enormous. This would be a way of developing an institution that is not autonomous but rather diffused and rooted in the community.

Finally, the present model of healthcare is increasingly tilted toward the *wealthy.* An alternative model of medical science should be tilted toward the *poor,* those who make up the majority of the human race.[5]

Table 2 lists some contrasting principles that might have strategic bearing on the Catholic healthcare apostolate's future:

TABLE 2: MODELS OF MEDICAL SCIENCE	
Modern	Postmodern
Reactive	Preventive
Specialized	Holistic
Technocratic	Participatory
Management	Creativity
Hospital focused	Community focused
Wealthy	Poor of the earth

I will close with three short-term, suggestions on how to begin pursuing such a vision.

Conclusion

First, *trust the laity's spiritual power.* This is first a message to members of religious communities who have been trained not to think that way. Also, this is a message to the laity, who often overlook their spiritual gifts, as if such gifts belong only to some specialized group. We must trust the laity's spiritual power and begin to reorient our thinking accordingly. The laity are not, of course, to be formed in the model of spirituality that shaped the modern religious orders. They must allow a spirituality to grow out of their own experience. This spirituality will give energy and new life to the healthcare apostolate.

Second, *commit to a long-range, reflection process.* The ideas I offer here may or may not be serviceable. They may or may not be right. But we are on the verge of a very different period of history and of an acute social crisis. One of the most important ways of unleashing creativity is to create a space for imaginative energies to work, not simply to allow ourselves to be absorbed into the day-to-day management of affairs. Management remains important, but management must be supplemented by room for reflection and creativity.[6] Consider keeping places in your networks where that process can be nurtured, places where ongoing input, communal conversation, and common searching can go on.

Third, *establish within your systems some point of responsibility,* a desk or an office, for probing the question of creative futures for healthcare systems. Try to have at least one person, perhaps a team of people, who could become expert on the alternative experiments around the country and the world. There are a variety of experiments in new forms of social organization, new health paradigms, and so on. This desk or office could function as an antenna to discover seeds of creativity and to share them with the whole healthcare system for evaluation and feedback. Thus there might develop an inventory of visions and of practical concrete steps leading to long-range transformation.

In summary, I have shared one interpretation of the profound social and religious crisis of our civilization and of its impact on the Catholic health apostolate. The social system is in profound crisis, suggesting that the modern healthcare system's economic foundation is being undermined from the public and private sides and that the model of technological progress that uproots values and dissolves community is leading the healthcare system away from serving the general population. The religious order that has been the source of vision and of key personnel for the Catholic healthcare apostolate is also in crisis, requiring a new and supplementary source of religious energy. The laity is the energy source that will sustain and deepen the system's commitment to the poor in a time of trial.

We need a new model of social organization to sustain this commitment, one that does not draw primarily from the free market model of the Right or from the state-centered model of the Left. It must be a model of social organization that arises from a retrieval of the communitarian dimension of life through a renewal of the cooperative movement.

Finally, this new stage of the healthcare apostolate must incarnate itself in a postmodern paradigm of medical science, linking specialization with holism, reactive medicine with prevention, technology with participation, management with creativity and hospital with community and reaching out to the poor, the majority of the earth's population.

I believe that the Spirit of God is calling us to become a prophetic community challenging our surrounding secular culture's destructive logic by searching for an alternative healthcare system founded first (but not only) on the needs of the poor.[7] Catholic healthcare has begun that search. We need the grace of God for the courage and creativity to complete it.

Footnotes
1. This chapter sketches the main lines of the contemporary social crisis affecting healthcare.
2. It seems to me that the repression of the Polish workers, "Solidarity" organization is precisely a fruit of this new stage as Poland began rapidly to engage in the world market system.
3. For example, a few years ago the Canadian Film Board produced films about nuclear war and acid rain. The U.S. government was displeased that they were being imported. The U.S. Justice Department asked the Canadian government to notify it of every librarian and teacher who rented the films so that their names and addresses could be put into a computer databank of suspicious persons.

4. Note that many forms of social organization in the life of the West have grown out of religious experiments. For example, democracy grew in part out of the Dominican constitutions. Thomas Jefferson studied the organizational model of the Dominican religious order to understand how to create a democratic republic. Religion is not on the margin of society. At times, religion even pioneers the new forms of social history.

5. For more on this issue, see Chapter 10 "Generating a Truly *Catholic* Response in Difficult Times."

6. Maria Riley, OP, and James E. Hug, SJ, have developed one such participative reflection process for healthcare institutions and systems. Called *Leadership for Justice*, it includes video tapes and written material to facilitate (1) analysis of the structural dimensions of experience in the light of religious faith and (2) planning for a more effective faith-filled response of the contemporary social crisis. More information on the program is available from the Center of Concern, Washington, DC.

7. For more on this theme, see Chapter 5, "Services of the Poor: The Foundation of Judeo-Christian Response."

Reflection Questions

1. This chapter's basic thesis is that our civilization is experiencing a profound social and religious transformation. In the midst of this turbulence, we are called to be people of faith, open to the possibility of change and future fulfillment.
   - What creative forces for this change do you detect in the current healthcare milieu? What destructive forces? What ambiguous forces?
   - What ways are available for the healthcare community to respond appropriately? For you personally to respond?
2. The chapter indicates that in this age of national security, governments will redesign their nations to make their countries attractive investment opportunities for transnational capital. Consumers, the state, and employers all will have less money to spend on healthcare services. This retrenchment of funds will create severe strains on healthcare providers.
   - What is being done in your area to heighten people's awareness of what is happening?
   - What more can be done?
3. Catholic healthcare systems were founded on the model of religious orders. They were envisioned to provide for the needs of God's people in a quasisocial welfare state.
   - Can Catholic healthcare systems deal with the new lay model, built on men and women, married and single with short-term, medium-term, and lifelong commitments, forming a pluralistic community of many styles? Give reasons for your answer.
   - What new ways do you envision through which Catholic healthcare providers can further life and health apart from the institutional settings with which we are familiar?
   - How could these new ways unleash new sources of energy?
4. Religious congregations model a unique form of private, collective ownership.
   - Is this model worth exploring as an example of the way(s) individuals can organize into groups to promote the common good? Give reasons for your answer.

5. This chapter proposes that in shaping the future we must (1) trust the laity's spiritual power, (2) engage in a long-term reflective process, and (3) allow space for creative energies to work.
   - What is your felt response to these considerations? Explain.
   - Would you qualify or take exception to any of these principles? Which? Why or why not?
   - What can you do to further the implementation or adoption of these principles?

Toward Healing Healthcare

As Catholic healthcare works to clarify its sense of identity and dedicates itself to discerning God's activity and invitation in our contemporary experience, many rich opportunities for transformative action exist. Section IV explores a few of these opportunities in search of steps that must be taken today and tomorrow to heal our society and our healthcare system.

Chapters 8 and 9 raise the neuralgic issue of labor unions in Catholic healthcare. Chapter 8 sets the question in a broad historical context, warning that fighting against unions in our institutions could repeat the mistake that cost the church the working class in the 19th century. It reminds us of the support for unions in Catholic social teaching, examines some of the principal arguments against unions, and explores the possibility of some new creative relationships between management and labor. It suggests that unions could become resources in the development of the type of alternative healthcare system the nation needs, and ends with some practical suggestions sure to stimulate discussion.

Chapter 9 explores Catholic social teaching on unions and on work much more extensively. From that teaching it develops guidelines for management, unions, and the public at large. It calls us to ground our responses in the sense of vocation that should be at the heart of healthcare employees' work.

A stark assessment of the situation of healthcare ministry in the United States opens Chapter 10. It celebrates and encourages U.S. Catholic healthcare institutions' and systems' commitment to the U.S. poor and proceeds to challenge them to expand their vision and recognize their responsibility for the global poor. It raises some important questions about U.S. culture, and it invites us to embrace the sense of the universal family of God that is at the heart of true Catholicism.

How can the church influence this somewhat grim economic situation in healthcare? Chapter 11 looks to *Economic Justice for All: Pastoral Letter on Catholic Social Teaching and the U.S. Economy* for some guidelines. It sees potential influence through the process by which the letter was developed, the analysis it offers of the economic and cultural forces at work in the United States today, its interpretation of these forces in the light of Christian faith and tradition, and finally the integrity with which all church institutions—especially healthcare institutions—model the justice the letter calls for. Some of the specific suggestions are quite controversial and challenging.

The final chapter interprets the current situation as part of a major global transition, the changing of an era. It encourages those who give pastoral care—and all of us—to become more aware of the social dimensions of the ministry we offer and of the divine revelation and call to conversion that they carry. It points out parallels between the current U.S. experience and the experience of ancient Israel at the time of the Babylonian Exile, and it explores the challenges that this situation presents for how we do our ministry. How can the way we serve in ministry help usher in a more just global order?

· 8 ·

The Call
for a Prophetic Healthcare System[1]

Joe Holland

If the question of unions in Catholic healthcare facilities is approached narrowly as a management issue with guidance taken from conventional secular wisdom, the result will be great damage to the Catholic healthcare ministry's evangelizing thrust and its creative possibilities as a prophetic alternative. Rather, the question must be approached broadly. This certainly means dealing with the church's social teaching on labor, but it means more. It requires placing the question within an analysis of the contemporary social crisis (including the related crisis of the healthcare system) and within correlative reflection on the changing form of the church's strategy for evangelization (including the relation of the Catholic healthcare ministry to it). These two frames—analysis of the social context and of the new directions in evangelization—provide the background against which to set this crucial moral and organizational issue.

Pursuing the question of unions in Catholic facilities against this background will fundamentally challenge the operating styles of both management and unions within Catholic healthcare. It will suggest that both Catholic management and unions must cooperate to create a prophetic Catholic health system based on an alternative model of healthcare that responds to the evangelical commitment to the preferential option for the poor.

120

I should also say here that creating such a prophetic Catholic healthcare system would move the debate beyond the liberal-conservative alternatives of central government planning versus free enterprise medicine. Both polarities are pushing the Catholic healthcare system away from its prophetic call. Rather than being organized on the politically bureaucratic governmental model or on the economically ruthless free enterprise model, Catholic healthcare is called to reroot itself prophetically in community.

Before exploring that, however, let us review the new social context and the shifting strategy for evangelization, within which the contemporary question of management-labor relations in Catholic healthcare institutions surfaces.

The New Social and Ecclesial Context

The overall social context within which modern healthcare arises and contemporary management-labor conflicts emerge is industrial society in general and, for America, industrial capitalism.

Stages in the Developing Context

Before the Industrial Revolution, modern social apostolates such as ministries in health, education, and other charitable works were limited phenomena in church and society.[2] The social dislocation of the Industrial Revolution led to the birth of many new religious congregations. Heroic women and men (more often women) were moved by great compassion at the sight of a disrupted peasantry cast from their rural roots into the heartless world of the new urban industrial centers. They looked around, saw the suffering of the unemployed, orphaned, homeless, and ill, and acted in spontaneous and direct ministries. They cared for the orphans, sheltered the homeless, nursed the sick, and taught the illiterate. They did not act solely as individuals; in the midst of their ministries, they called others to join them. Thus were born the modern activist religious congregations, dedicated to social service for the poor.

Many of the European hierarchy were disturbed by these new religious movements, as they were by the modern world in general. They tried to defend the church against the modern world and to prevent the emergence of these new orders. It was a conflict paralleling the ancient one between Peter and Paul: Should the church preach to the Gentiles or remain only with the Jews? Should the church reach out to the modern world or retreat into a ghetto? Although many of the bishops were building the walls of the Catholic ghetto, the new religious were already reaching out to the victims of the modern world.

In the United States, new religious orders either came from abroad or were born here after the great industrial expansion that began in 1840. Immigrants poured in by the millions to work the mines, mills, and factories. They came to a society with few nurses, physicians, or hospitals. They were poor, underpaid, and often abandoned in illness or injury both by employers and by government. Into this context came the new religious, again mainly women, as their only solace. Thus, in early industrial society the face of Jesus often appeared to the sick poor in the image of sisters.

These new religious congregations began their work in the disruptive and harsh context of early industrial capitalism. Their ministries were spontaneous, direct, and rooted in communities of ordinary people. Often these ministers were not well educated, but their zeal more than made up for any educational shortcomings. The great Catholic social institutions that exist today (hospitals, schools, and orphanages) are a continuing testimony to ordinary people's power to change the world.

This early period of industrial capitalism, concentrated in the 19th century, has been called the *laissez faire* period. The most outrageous example of *laissez faire* was the Irish famine of the mid-19th century, where the British government held that it had no public responsibility to help the starving Irish peasantry when their potato crop failed. While potatoes (the crop of the poor) failed, other crops owned by the great plantations and destined for export flourished. As a result, the problem was left to be "solved" by free market forces, with the resulting death or emigration of half the population.

In the 20th century, however, a new period of industrial capitalism took shape, namely, the social welfare period. During this time, government intervened dramatically in the economy, especially on the poor's behalf, and Catholic social service

ministries became institutions. On the one hand, this led to public social welfare institutions that competed with Catholic ones.
On the other hand, it led to the incorporation of Catholic social
welfare ministries into the heart of a revised church strategy for
evangelization. Thus, while during the 19th century the official
evangelization strategy rejected the modern world, during the 20th
century the church competed with the secular modern world precisely on the terrain of social welfare institutions.

These Catholic social welfare institutions, which never
before existed on such a scale, can be described as parallel structures. They parallel the main forms of socialization within the
industrial society. As parallel structures, they served two key functions in addition to their immediate task: (1) to compete with their
secular parallels for the loyalty of the Catholic people and so to
provide defensive social environments where Catholic social
principles could be protected while integrating the Catholic community into the modern world; and (2) to provide bases of
influence for the church in the wider society. This reorganization
of the church's strategy for evangelization around parallel structures marked a basic strategic shift.

During the *laissez faire* period, the church's dominant and
official strategy could be described as traditionalist. It rejected the
modern world and tried to organize its resources to protect tradition against the modern world. To enter the modern world would
threaten tradition, no matter how many persons would be helped.
But during the social welfare period, thanks in part to the work
of these pioneering religious, the church adopted a strategy of
cautious integration into the modern world. This can be described
as a liberal strategy, not in the sense of liberalizing the church
internally, but of accommodating the church to the liberal environment. The new Catholic social services, emerging as major institutional networks, provided the foundation and leading edge of that
new strategy.

But it was not only the church that changed; society had
changed too. Industrial capitalism grew more benevolent, with
increasing public and private concern for health, education, and
welfare. Eventually, a federal cabinet-level department focused on
these themes emerged. But even more important, the harsh and
exploitative period of industrial capitalism had passed for many.

Children and grandchildren of 19th century industrial immigrants were now more prosperous—receiving good salaries, working in better conditions, buying houses and cars, and sending their children to college. In sum, the American Catholic immigrant church produced a substantial middle class. And with this change, the institutional social service ministries took a more middle-class character.

The healthcare institutions accepted modern organizational techniques and objectives. Both acute and long term care facilities developed larger complexes, more advanced technology, greater medical specialization, and contemporary management styles taken from major business schools. Eventually they hired large staffs in management, medicine, nursing, and supportive services. In fact, the Catholic healthcare ministry has become one the largest social service employers in the country.

In this context, as healthcare costs rose, the costs were covered for the more affluent by private insurance programs and for at least some of the poor by government welfare programs. Thus, even though the Catholic healthcare system had begun in a context in which the sick were often abandoned both by employers and by government and left to voluntary charity, the tables were turned. Big business (insurance) and big government (welfare) paid the bills, and church institutions acted as channels for service. Eventually, however, a series of interrelated crises marked the end of the benevolent social welfare period and produced a shift in the church's evangelization as well. These shifts, too complex to analyze here, are leading to a general social crisis of which the particular crisis in healthcare is but one part.[3]

The same series of interrelated crises has produced a shift in the church's evangelization as well. There is now need for a more prophetic Catholic strategy for evangelization and, hence, for a prophetic Catholic healthcare system.

The Contemporary Context

In the new period of social history, sometimes referred to as the national security period, the majority of the American people may suffer long term economic hardship. On the one hand, business will no longer provide the reward for labor that it did in the social welfare period. Rather, living standards are already moving from prosperity toward a new austerity. For the majority of Americans, this already means the receding of the "American dream." The majority may no longer be able to afford a house, a car, or a college education for their children.

At the same time, there are new attacks on the one instrument that can defend the rights of the working majority of the country, namely, unions. These attacks come from the media, from government, and from management. Some in the media portray unions as racist, corrupt, and too powerful. Nonetheless they may be one of the better integrated institutions in the country, less corrupt than business, although often weak. Government, increasingly shaped by neoconservative offensives, is attempting to undercut much of the prolabor legislation constructed since the New Deal of Franklin Roosevelt. Finally, management, which a decade ago often accepted unions in principle, has now developed a new antiunion approach that stresses management's prerogatives. Salaries continue to decline under inflation, and in many cases workers must work longer hours, at faster rates, or on several jobs just to break even.

Government is now backing away from its social welfare role, stressing instead deregulation of the economy and curtailing social spending while expanding military spending. In coming years we will probably see reduction or termination of programs such as Social Security, Unemployment Compensation, Aid to Families with Dependent Children, Medicare, and Medicaid.

There is not space here to explain the structural roots of the new situation. Suffice it to say that because capital is now international and technology so capital intensive, all nations are forced to redesign their internal social systems radically to provide competitive investment environments in the world market system. This leads to pressures to (1) lower wages (often by breaking or forbidding unions), (2) lower taxes (by dropping social spending), (3) increase militarization (to guarantee access to strategic resources like oil, provide secure shipping and marketing abroad, and protect foreign investments), and (4) impose political stability (by suppressing dissent, either by direct force or by political manipulation).[4] Figure 1 illustrates the shifting contexts of healthcare ministry.

Looking at the church globally in this new context, one

125

sees a new prophetic strategy for evangelization taking shape. In the *laissez faire* context, the church was split between an officially traditionalist strategy and the new direct social ministries of new religious orders. In the social welfare context, the church adopted a liberal strategy centered on parallel structures (e.g., hospitals and schools) as defensive and integrating instruments. Now, in the new national security context, the church is beginning to redesign its ministries around the prophetic task of defending the poor.

This new strategy includes the positive task of constructing new alternatives in healthcare, education, and a variety of other arenas to serve and defend the poor's basic needs and fundamental rights.

In this new strategy, the church is led to a prophetic encounter with the wider society—not simply to adapt itself to the modern world, but to transform it. The leading theme in this context becomes "faith and justice." The preaching of the Gospel is intimately bound up with defense of the poor. In this new strategy, the key task is to form basic Christian communities, especially among the poor, since they provide the seeds of a new society and a renewed church.

The church often pays a great price for this prophetic role, as did Jesus. A new wave of persecution is spreading across the church in some areas of the world, as Christians are once again condemned for being subversive and are imprisoned, tortured, exiled, and even martyred.

What is the relevance of this discussion for Catholic healthcare or for the management-labor relationships within it? This brings us to our second major heading: the implications of the new social context and evangelizing strategy for Catholic healthcare.

Implications for Catholic Healthcare

It is no longer sufficient to maintain a parallel Catholic structure operating on the same medical model as the wider secular healthcare system. Why? Because the convergence of crises is pressing the healthcare system away from serving the poor toward an increasingly expensive, technocratic, and, in some ways, ineffective healthcare system.

FIGURE 1: SUMMARY OF THE SHIFTING CONTEXTS OF HEALTHCARE MINISTRY		
SOCIAL CONTEXT	ECCLESIAL CONTEXT	FORM OF MINISTRY
Laissez Faire Stage 19th Century	Traditionalist Catholic strategy, pre-modern institutions	Preinstitutional healthcare ministry, direct and spontaneous
Social Welfare Stage: Early and Mid 20th Century	Liberal Catholic strategy, modern institutions as parallel structures	Parallel institutional healthcare ministry, modeled on dominant system
National Security: Late 20th Century	Prophetic Catholic strategy, alternative structures	Alternative institutional healthcare ministry, based on option for the poor

The new austerity may mean that the majority of Americans will be reluctant to use healthcare except in very serious cases, simply because they cannot afford it. Insurance becomes ever more expensive for the middle class, paralleling the rise in health-care costs, and leaves much uncovered. Welfare is being dismantled, leaving the poor unprotected. The only people with adequate support for health services will be the affluent minority. This may seem an exaggerated prognosis, but it is the direction in which the American healthcare system is pointed.

Thus, Catholic healthcare, if it continues on its present trajectory, could wind up the very opposite of what it was originally intended to be—not an evangelical mission serving those abandoned by society, but a nonevangelical institution reflecting secular logic, rejecting the abandoned, and serving the affluent.

I should quickly add that I do not believe that this will happen. I believe that those who preside over Catholic healthcare have the faith and commitment to search for more creative alternatives.

The Search for Alternatives

The search for alternatives will mean moving beyond reliance either on central state planning and subsidies or on free-market mechanisms. One would withdraw support from the poor; the other would exclude the poor outright; and both would reinforce the dominant technocratic style. Rather, the key resources will come from *ordinary people in rooted community, searching for alternatives in healthcare to meet their basic needs.*

In general, an alternative to our current healthcare system will have to shift its main operating assumptions. The present healthcare system can be described as increasingly reactive, specialized, technocratic, and exclusionary. The alternative system we need should be preventive, holistic, participatory, and all-encompassing.

To think such alternative thoughts becomes an imperative as the church reorganizes its strategy for evangelization around the preferential option for the poor. But with such thoughts, *Catholic healthcare's key task is to focus not on management, but rather on creativity.* The task is not simply to manage what *is*, but to create what *is not yet.* If this creative task seems beyond our ability, we have only to recall the creative faith of the simple women and men who built Catholic healthcare; they were anything but realists.

In seeking to be faithful to their foundational charisms, our contemporary task is neither to repeat what they did (spontaneous, direct, noninstitutional ministry) nor to perpetuate what their successors built (a parallel Catholic institutional healthcare system). It is rather to redesign Catholic healthcare, with its institutional strength, into a prophetic and alternative system organized around the preferential option for the poor.

This means that we must begin to speak of *prophetic institutions.* Normally, we think of prophets as persons who reject institutions. Many of the more prophetic persons in religious congregations with a healthcare ministry have rejected the institutional forms of ministry and returned to the direct service more typical of their founders or foundresses. But although such individual witness is often heroic, is it sufficient or even desirable to abandon the institutional apparatus that in the long run may be of much greater service to the poor than countless individual ministries? It is a wonderful thing for individual health ministers to work directly with the poor. But how much greater it would be if committed individuals could turn the whole direction of Catholic healthcare.

It is perhaps also easier for prophetic religious individuals not to address the complex problems right in their own backyard. Thus, we see in religious congregations today great concern for the poor in Latin America or Appalachia, but not always for poor employees in the institutions of their own congregations. Similarly, there is growing concern for the rights of women in the church, but is there also attention to the rights of registered and licensed practical nurses, ward secretaries, and other staff in Catholic healthcare facilities? There is danger here of the same dualism that has always infected the church in its social mission—concern for those outside, but not for those inside (Figure 2).

FIGURE 2: CONTRAST OF HEALTHCARE MINISTRIES' UNDERLYING MODELS		
Perspective	Dominant Model	Alternative Model
Temporal axis	Reactive	Preventive
Spacial axis	Specialized	Holistic
Governance	Technocratic	Participatory
Constituency	Favors the rich	Option for poor
Key virtue	Management	Creativity

The Question of Unions

Are unions an obstacle or a resource for Catholic healthcare ministry? Let me pose two distinct ways of addressing this question. On the one hand, *if the issue of unions is addressed from a framework that assumes that the present healthcare system is good, then unions will appear as a threat to its security.* On the other hand, *if the issue of unions is addressed from a framework that assumes that an alternative healthcare system is needed, then unions could become a resource.* These two ways of addressing the question need more discussion.

In the first case, we assume that Catholic healthcare is on the right track in simply copying the technological and financial models of the wider society. But the healthcare system is experiencing serious strains. Consider the following:

- Costs of providing care are rising astronomically, while personal income is still limited.
- Hospitals have often expanded over the years, making them much larger enterprises than previously envisioned. Because of the complexity and financial expansion of healthcare and because of the shortage of trained members of religious communities, governance of the healthcare institution is increasingly entrusted to secular or lay specialists.
- The path of medicine and health in general is shaped by physicians, trained for long years at the cost of hundreds of thousands of dollars. These specialists in turn have grown into a class apart, living in a medical subculture and isolated further by the fact that their class is one of the wealthiest in the country.
- Financial decisions are shaped by high level business people who sit on boards of directors and are generally extremely wealthy (usually men). Of course they are not on boards because they are greedy—just the opposite. They are there to help the institutions, and they give abundantly of their time and expertise—often with no reward except the personal satisfaction of knowing they have contributed to a good cause.
- Next, management is entrusted to lay people—sometimes Catholic, sometimes not. These people are trained in modern methods of secular management, perhaps at general business schools, but more often at specialized schools adapting general business training to healthcare institutions. These people normally have not been given any special training in the tradition of Catholic social thought or in the long history of the religious congregation's encounter with the modern world. It is assumed that their secular technical skills alone equip them for the task of management.

- Finally, when difficult problems arise, outside guidance is widely available from law firms or management consulting groups who have developed particular expertise in these difficult areas.

In sum, there has been a fundamental reversal in the nature of the leadership presiding over Catholic healthcare. What was begun for the most part by religious women in direct ministry to the poor is now presided over mainly by rich, secularly competent men trying to protect healthcare institutions' economic security.

Most often, these technical experts' motives and dedication are superior to those of the general population. But they take their orientation from the conventional secular wisdom of cost-accounting techniques. As such, they steer the healthcare system in a particular direction, one modeled on the modern business corporation.

Then, along comes a union! Perhaps the employees have some legitimate grievances that have not been attended to. Perhaps the union organizer is only fishing. In any case, the union is there and the alarm sounds. The sponsoring community immediately become frightened. It has little experience in this area and so turns to the "experts." The board members, mainly business people, see unions as an enemy that cuts into profit margins. The physicians, one of the last examples of the successful independent entrepreneur, have little use for social solidarity and also see unions as the enemy—corrupt, money hungry, too powerful, and disruptive of the healthcare workplace. The managers, often trained in new antiunion management styles, feel their authority is being undermined and see the union as the enemy. They all seek help from law firms or management consultants.

In some cases the union's presence may be unwarranted, and it is easily defeated. Other cases may be more ambiguous, and a struggle ensues. In still other cases the employees may really want a union, and a bitter polarization occurs. In this case, the institution is marked with deep scars that may last for decades.

Whatever the situation, the judgment is presided over by the upper classes of society—board members, managers, physicians, lawyers, and consultants. The church is increasingly seeing the world through the poor's eyes, while the hospital is making decisions from the wealthy's perspective.

The same thing happened in Europe in the 19th century, when unions first arose. The church viewed the question originally through the eyes of the rich—not then the rich technical specialists, but the rich landed aristocracy. To them, unions were a rebellion against the divine order of rich and poor and therefore the enemy. Most of the leaders of the European church accepted this frame of reference, and ordinary people—working people—came to see the church as their enemy. As a result, in those areas where the European labor movement gained strength, it was forced to fight the church. Many workers gave up being Catholic. The loss of the industrial working class in the European church was the greatest pastoral tragedy of the 19th century. Why did it happen? Because the church read the situation through the eyes of the rich and not the poor.

The same thing is happening again, although the rich are no longer the landed aristocracy. Today they control technical expertise and define the shape of our social system and its sub-systems. Once again we are seeing a new labor movement being born—not in the industrial sector but in the service sector, not in Europe but in America. As this labor movement arises, gathering constituencies among acute and long term care facilities' workers, it shows itself to be a complex movement. Some organizers are ethical, others are not. Sometimes employees want the union, sometimes they do not. The union's actual behavior is not the deepest question. The deepest question is, rather, how the management of the Catholic healthcare system views the unions. Frequently it views them as the enemy. Thus, it repeats the pattern of the 19th century European church and jeopardizes the very loyalty of workers to the U.S. church. That loyalty was once our special hallmark and the foundation for a successful model of evangelization.

Destructive Attitudes

In this process, several rationalizations arise to justify the view of the union as the enemy of the Catholic healthcare mission.

First, it is sometimes argued that the Catholic institution, because it is religious, differs from the rest of the work world. It is claimed to be modeled on the Christian family, whereas the rest of society is not. But any honest examination from a sociological viewpoint would disclose that, in fact, a Catholic hospital is usually very much the same as a secular hospital. It differs only in having a different sponsoring group, some religious services, and in judging certain medical practices immoral. But the structure and style of management—that is, the nature of employer-employee relationships—is no different. Indeed, antiunion Catholic management and antiunion secular management cooperate.

Hence, this claim to be different becomes a smokescreen for authoritarian relationships between management and labor. This is particularly ironic, since religious congregations have been busy ever since Vatican II discarding authoritarian models of governance from their own internal congregational life. Nonetheless, they have continued to impose them on their own employees.

A second argument often proposed is that the union is an outside third party that destroys the intimacy of the employer-employee relationship by driving a wedge between the two. But this argument overlooks the fact that the relationship is already encumbered on the employer's side by multiple third parties who have destroyed the direct and intimate character of this relationship. They are management itself (as distinct from ownership or sponsorship), boards of directors (who probably never meet most of the employees yet set policy for them), management schools that set the style of dealing with employees, and law firms and specialized consultants that are hired (often at great expense) to shape management strategy *vis a vis* employees. Thus, on one side are the sponsors, the board, the management, university management schools, management associations, law firms, and consulting firms—a complex array of third parties. On the other side are the employees who stand alone. Should they desire a union, it would be nothing more than providing themselves with some of the same resources already assembled on the employer's side—legal support, educational resources, and organizational strength.

A third argument, framed in response to the undeniable fact that Catholic social teaching has been basically prounion since the late 19th century, argues that although unions were once good and necessary, they have outlived their usefulness. Today, it is argued, they are too corrupt and too strong or else no longer necessary because of the new "participatory" management styles (e.g., open-door policies).

The first response to this argument could easily be to observe how strange it is that no one has told Pope John Paul II of this change. Defending the rights of employees to organize, free of harassment, has been one of his main social themes. His encyclical on the rights of labor, *On Human Work (Laborem Exercens)*, refers to unions as an "indispensable element of social life."[5] Obviously, no one told the Polish workers about this either, although communist governments make the same claim as some of Catholic management against independent unions, namely, that they disrupt society or institutions and that participation is already guaranteed.

In fact, just the opposite could be argued, namely, that unions may be more necessary than ever and also may be weaker than ever. Precisely because American society is entering into a deep social crisis, there is the danger of trying to solve the problems of the healthcare institutions at the expense of the employees and the poor. But just the reverse is called for—not to exclude people from participation in decisions to solve problems, but to broaden the participation of ordinary people in the basic decision-making processes precisely to guarantee that the solutions will be creative and human.

Thus, in this first way of solving the question of unions, the negative direction of the healthcare system and the authoritarian social control over it is reinforced. The institution begins to read the society and its healthcare problems through the eyes of the rich rather than the poor. Unions are seen as enemies of management or as obstacles to defending the institutional security of the present form of healthcare. This response, besides deepening the crisis of the healthcare system, contributes to a breakdown of evangelization by the U.S. Catholic church, since it threatens to repeat the de-Christianization of labor that happened in 19th century Europe.

An Alternative Approach

The second way of responding to the question of unions would require that it be tied to the possibility of an alternative healthcare system. In this case, the union might become a resource rather than an obstacle. If a Catholic healthcare institution is faced with a deepening fiscal crisis and perhaps even with closing, management does not have to deal with the crisis alone. The employees are involved as well. Perhaps some union representatives are already on the board of directors of the institution, or perhaps they simply have good working relationships with management, developed in a cooperative and open bargaining spirit.

Labor and management together, then, could face the question of the institution's future. Both might agree they want the hospital to survive and even to improve its service to the community in general and the poor in particular. New forms of cooperative management might be developed that could dramatically increase productivity. New forms of healthcare and technology might be developed to enable low-income people to get better access to healthcare services at lower costs. For example, an extensive program of paraprofessionals could be developed, as well as new forms of outreach such as home-delivery midwife programs. The hospital might reorient its philosophy around a wellness concept in health and develop community education programs in nutrition and disease prevention. New cooperative forms of payment might be explored, such as the health maintenance organization (HMO). In addition, the union, with its extensive educational and lobbying apparatus, could develop new cost-cutting policies and gain community and governmental support for them. Under union supervision, day-care services might be provided for employees and a network of neighborhood clinics developed.

Suggestions for the Future

I would like to offer some practical transitional guidelines to help bring such an alternative vision into reality:

1. Begin a "precrisis" dialogue with labor. A national forum for dialogue is needed between the sponsors and managers of Catholic healthcare and the leaders of unions active in this area. The focus of this dialogue must move beyond the "prerogatives

of management." It also needs to move beyond a narrow self-understanding of union's role. It is wrong to see unions only in an adversarial relationship with management, letting management worry about how to make ends meet and about the nature of the healthcare system and having the union only concerned with employee wages and benefits. Rather, the focus of the dialogue should be management's and labor's common concern for a creative, sustainable, and just healthcare system. If such a dialogue were to develop, I believe unions would appear much more an ally than an enemy.

2. Boards of directors should be microcosms of their communities. If the healthcare system is to move in a prophetic direction, the nature of the boards of directors must shift. They should no longer be made up only of "technical experts" from business and medicine. They should reflect the wider community and include representatives from the labor movement in the area, perhaps some elected employee representatives, and major health-care consumers such as the elderly, the handicapped, and the poor. The poor in particular should have a privileged place on boards. It will, of course, be argued that the issues that boards address are too complex for "ordinary people," but just the opposite is true. What is at stake is shaping the fundamental values of the health-care system—something too important to leave to experts and to the wealthy.

3. Lay management needs the support of sustained Christian formation. Although in recent years religious congregations have benefited from extensive education about the church's growing commitment to the poor, lay managers are often hired for their technical competence. The sponsors must develop for these lay managers extensive training programs in the church's new social orientation and in the background of Catholic social thought. In addition, where new management is being selected, Gospel values of commitment to the poor and an understanding of democratic management as a form of Christian ministry should be criteria for selection.

4. Management should increasingly be modeled on the management structures of cooperatives. Presently management models are taken from secular business schools, but Catholic healthcare institutions are much more than secular businesses. It

would be well, therefore, to explore the alternative management model carried by the cooperative movement, to which the church has been deeply committed in the past.

5. Lawyers should be consulted within carefully defined limits. The United States is now the most lawyer-encumbered nation in the world, with the courts becoming the place where social questions are resolved. Unfortunately, this undermines the social fabric and is extremely expensive. The legal profession has a vested interest in adversary relationships, whether they be management lawyers or labor lawyers. Instead, we need to find new, less legalistic, and more cooperative ways to resolve conflicts. Especially, we need to beware of letting lawyers expand their competence unduly. Technical expertise in legal matters does not qualify them as master strategists for relating with unions. Lawyers should be prepared to explain what legal consequences a given course of action entails, but the sponsors must set the course.

6. Define the health mission around the preferential option for the poor. Since Vatican II, the 1971 Synod of Bishops, and the meetings of the Latin American Bishops at Medellin and Puebla, there has been a growing orientation of the Catholic church's pastoral thrust toward the poor. The 1986 The Catholic Health Association study, *No Room in the Marketplace,* and the efforts of several health systems are encouraging signs that this orientation is making its presence felt in healthcare.[6] It should be the defining principle around which ministry is eventually organized. This is a very different principle, by the way, than is normally mediated by management schools or legal advisers. It requires long strategic planning and gradual shifting of institutional directions.

In conclusion, the coming decade of Catholic healthcare will be one of searching reappraisal. It will probably also be marked by increasing conflicts over underlying social and religious values. But I have little doubt that out of this conflict will come a new and deepening commitment to an evangelical and prophetic healthcare system, organized around the preferential option for the poor. As this happens, I also believe that unions (made up mostly of poor healthcare workers) will be considered an enemy no longer, but a friend.

Footnotes
1. This chapter is a revision of an article by Joe Holland, *"The Labor-Management Dialogue: Church Perspectives,"* Adam J. Maida, ed., The Catholic Health Association, St. Louis, 1982.
2. For more on these themes see Chapter 7, "The Sociomedical History: A Look at the Forces Shaping the Contemporary Context."
3. See Chapter 7, "The Sociomedical History: A Look at the Forces Shaping the Contemporary Context."
4. See Chapter 7, "The Sociomedical History: A Look at the Forces Shaping the Contemporary Context."
5. Pope John Paul II, *On Human Work*, #20, *Origins*, vol. 11, no. 15, Sept. 24, 1981, pp. 239-240.
6. *No Room in the Marketplace: Health Care of the Poor* (Final Report of The Catholic Health Association's Task Force on Health Care of the Poor), The Catholic Health Association of the United States, St. Louis, 1986. Several health systems have done their own studies, including, for example, Mercy Health Services and The Bon Secours Health System.

Reflection Questions

1. Describe the effects of "benevolent capitalism" and an increasing public and private concern for social services on Catholic healthcare institutions.

2. This chapter states that in this national security period, governments will radically redesign their internal social systems to provide a competitive environment in the world market system. To do this they will lower wages, lower taxes, increase militarization, and impose political stability.
   - What signs do you see of this strategy?
   - What are the effects of governmental constraints on healthcare today? In your institution(s)?
   - How can the church redesign its ministry of healthcare to become a better model of service that is preventive, holistic, participatory, and encompassing?
   - How might your institution(s) play a prophetic role in the contemporary situation?

3. This chapter cites three rationalizations usually applied against unions: that a Catholic institution is different from the rest of the world; that a union is an outside, third party; and that unions have outlived their usefulness.
   - Do you find the opposing arguments—that in reality Catholic institutions are not substantially different from other institutions in their labor and management relations; that in the healthcare environment many third parties are already aligned with management; and that the Church has repeatedly and consistently defended the right of labor to organize convincing? Why?

4. The chapter describes the desired labor-management relationship as (1) broadening the participation of ordinary people, (2) having an openness to the possibility of alternative delivery systems, and (3) developing a cooperative and open bargaining spirit.
   - Can you see these dispositions as possibilities? Explain.
   - Do other obstacles militate against such a relationship being established? Explain.

· 9 ·

Unionization, The Call of the Church, and The Catholic Healthcare Institution[1]

Peter J. Henriot, SJ

I would like to begin by placing the topic of unionization and Catholic healthcare institutions in an historical perspective. The Catholic community worldwide has been irreversibly changed by the Second Vatican Council. The great document that ended the Council, indeed, the chief document of that Council, is *The Church in the Modern World*.

The Church in the Modern World resulted from an internal debate within the Council. The central question around which the debate swirled was: "Is it possible to speak about the modern church, its nature, its characteristics, its mission without speaking about the modern world and the signs of the times that people are increasingly aware of?" The Council declared very clearly from the first words of the document how the Christian community and the world that it is immersed in are related:

> The joys and the hopes, the griefs and the anxieties
> of the [women and] men of this age, especially those
> who are poor or in any way afflicted, these too are the
> joys and hopes, the griefs and anxieties of the followers
> of Christ.[2]

The world that we are in the midst of and the church that we are part of are integrally related. As we reflect on our call to serve today, we should remember that we must embrace those joys and hopes, griefs and anxieties if we want to be faithful followers of Jesus.

With this in mind, I would like to develop five major points demonstrating the relationship among unions, Catholic healthcare ministry, and the mission set forth by Vatican II. First, as the *context* for the question of unions, Catholic healthcare must recall the priority of the values of the "healthcare ministry" model over those of the "healthcare industry" model. Second, *the issue of unionization* in Catholic healthcare institutions at this critical juncture is being shaped by several important internal and external factors. Third, *Church teachings* offer strong challenging directives for dealing with the issue. Fourth, I want to suggest some practical *guidelines* for institutions, unions, and the general public to help in implementing the church's teaching. Finally, I believe it is important to highlight the *vocation* of people as the essential perspective working in Catholic healthcare institutions and the challenges facing them.

The Context of Catholic Healthcare

The future of U.S. Catholic healthcare is a widely debated topic. Its identity, direction, and conditions for survival are all very important subjects for discussion by those involved with Catholic healthcare institutions. The essays in this book all wrestle with various aspects of this future.

There is no need to review here the questions about unions raised in the previous chapter. However, I do believe it is important to remind ourselves as we approach the volatile issue of unions that Catholic healthcare must maintain its commitment to the model of healthcare ministry as its *primary* commitment. The values promoted by the healthcare industry model must be kept in service to those held up by the ministry model.

The healthcare ministry model, to summarize briefly, is characterized by (1) service of persons, reverencing the dignity of the individual in his or her social context; (2) a holistic approach serving the whole person in the relational context of her or his communities; (3) a focus on the spiritual, on that life force within the individual that animates and integrates all dimensions of bodily life; (4) cooperation for enrichment and mutuality in service; and (5) an option for the poor.[3] The healthcare industry model in contrast, is characterized by (1) a focus on marketing a product; (2) great attention to the margin of profit, the return on investment;

(3) an emphasis on specialization for the sake of efficiency; (4) an emphasis on technology; (5) a stress on competition; and (6) a commitment to growth for the sake of remaining competitive.[4]

Both sets of values are important, but it is essential that business values *serve* ministry values, not dominate or eclipse them.

The Issue of Unionization

As the issue of unionization is introduced, the question of industry and ministry models becomes even more complex. There are increasing efforts by a variety of unions to enroll workers in healthcare institutions. Unionization can occur in many different sectors, including housekeeping services, kitchen, maintenance, and nursing.

Why is the issue of unions becoming more part of the day-to-day life of U.S. healthcare? Two causal factors have been suggested—one internal, the other external.[5] The internal factor is a specific dynamic operative among healthcare institutions' employees that differs from that operative in many other businesses and institutions. The dynamic is known as a tier system. In most industries, there is room for advancement from the entry level positions. This is generally not the case in healthcare. Specialization keeps people in their particular "dead end" spots. In addition, recent studies have shown that employees at the lower levels of healthcare receive some of the lowest salaries for their skill levels in the business world. This generates a "seed-bed" for the entry of unions. In healthcare, then, unionization seems the only certain path to secure monetary advancement, since job advancement is unavailable.

External forces are also at work. Unions are becoming more aggressive in organizing nonunionized workers. Unions in the United States are on the defensive. Only 15 to 20 percent of U.S. workers are organized today. Unions are shrinking, mainly because some of the large industrial unions have seen their base eroded as steel mills and automobile factories closed. These traditional industries, once a stronghold for unions, have become smaller. As a result, unions are looking for new sources of membership, new businesses to organize. Healthcare seems an open and fertile field.

At the same time, healthcare institutions are facing

increasing financial constraints. Many are closing. Many are consolidating into systems. The environment is sharply competitive. If unions succeed in raising wages—and therefore increasing labor costs—they will appear a serious threat to an institution's competitiveness and consequent survival.

A third factor in this problematic is that many administrators view unions as outsiders, as troublemakers who come into an ordinarily placid situation and create unrest. Thus, they often feel that other outsiders must be brought in, management consultants who can advise management on how to ward off these unions.

Finally, this whole problem is compounded by the consistent church teaching that unions are important and workers should be organized. This is a central principle of Catholic social teaching, even though many Catholic hospital administrators have serious difficulties with it. This brings me to my third major point.

Church Teachings

The Center of Concern has published a small book on Catholic social teaching entitled *Catholic Social Teaching: Our Best Kept Secret.*[6] We chose that title because Catholic social teaching has been, in the United States at least, one of the least known elements of Catholic tradition.

This developing body of social wisdom has been influenced by the scriptures and by the teachings of early writers in the church, medieval philosophers, and theologians. Its major documents begin with *On the Condition of Labor (Rerum Novarum)* of Pope Leo XIII and continue in the work of Popes Pius XI, Pius XII, John XXIII, Paul VI, and John Paul II. Indeed, since the end of the Second Vatican Council, there has been a major flurry of Catholic social teaching.

Here in the United States, this teaching has been developed and expanded through pastoral letters from the bishops on such topics as human values, racism, nuclear arms and peace, the economy, and women's concerns. All this social teaching has a single purpose: to explore the challenge to live in the contemporary world as followers of Jesus sensitive to the joys and the hopes, the griefs, and the anxieties of our sisters and brothers, particularly those who are poor and in any way afflicted. That exploration has unearthed certain principles relating to work, workers, workers' associations, and institutions that employ workers. Let me briefly summarize those themes.

The Dignity of Work

First, Catholic social teaching highlights work's centrality and dignity. The encyclical letter of John Paul II, *On Human Work (Laborem Exercens),* begins:

> Through work, women and men must earn their daily bread and contribute to the continual advance of science and technology, and above all, to elevating increasingly the moral and cultural level of the society within which they live in community with all of those who make up the same human family.[7]

In the eyes of John Paul II, work is not only a way in which we earn our daily bread, it is the way in which we transform the society around us. Indeed, the theme developed in *On Human Work (Laborem Exercens)* is a constant theme in Catholic social teaching. Women and men, created in the image and likeness of God the creator, are cocreators with God. Our work is part of reality's ongoing creation and transformation. We continue that creation and transformation in relation to the earth and to each other.

The pastoral letter on the economy by the U.S. Catholic bishops, echoing John Paul II, points out that human work "has a special dignity and is key to achieving justice in society."[8] That is why unemployment is such a critical issue in our own country and, indeed, around the world. To deny people the opportunity to experience that they are made in the image and likeness of God the creator, is a blasphemy against the living God. Employment is central. Work is central. The dignity of work is central. That applies to all types of work: physical work, intellectual work, artistic work, administrative work, manual work, and housework. They are all part of our continuing, cocreative effort in the world.

That, then, is the first important principle of Catholic social teaching: the centrality and dignity of work.

Workers' Rights and Dignity

The second principle is the need to respect the rights and to protect the dignity of workers. Since 1891, when Leo XIII published the first major social encyclical, *On the Condition of Labor*

(Rerum Novarum), workers' rights and protection have been emphasized in Catholic social teaching.

John Paul II, in *On Human Work (Laborem Exercens),* developed that emphasis in a variety of ways. He insisted that we cannot understand work only in an objective sense. It is true that work is a product, an object produced, an activity that results in something. But that is not work's only or most important dimension. John Paul II reminded us that there is the subjective sense of work that exists because the human person is the subject of work. Work has a value because it is "my work," because it expresses me. A new car as a work of an industry has its value in human terms because humans worked on it.

Hence work, labor, is not a commodity to be bought and sold on the open market as steel would be to produce that car, or as coal, or energy would. Work is sacred because the worker is a human person. Hence labor—and this is John Paul II's teaching—always has priority over capital.

This priority of labor over capital does not mean that workers always have priority over managers who control the capital. It means that work, labor, and human effort expended always have priority over capital, money, and technological arrangements. We may look at an industry and admire its machines and high technology communications and control systems, but the more wonderful reality there is the unskilled person who attends to that machinery's operation. The dignity of work is rooted in the human person's dignity. This is at the heart of Catholic social teaching. That dignity must be respected and protected. That is why the issues of wages, working conditions, and rewards become central. Human persons are involved, and important conditions are required to nuture and protect their dignity. Providing these conditions is the employer's responsibility.

Pope John Paul II distinguishes between the direct employer and the indirect employer. The direct employer is the person or the institution providing the job. The indirect employer is the wider society, which conditions and shapes the situation within which work goes on. The government, public institutions, other business, households, and consumers are all "indirect employers" of workers.

The Role of Unions

The third point concerns the role of workers' associations or unions. Where work is of great dignity and workers respected, workers should be allowed to join associations to protect their basic dignity. Originally taught by Pope Leo XIII in 1891, this position is still put forward today in the church's social teaching. Pope John Paul II insists that workers' associations, unions, are indispensible elements of social life. They are not simply a "necessary evil" brought on by conflicts between workers and management—just the opposite. They are a "necessary good." They are part of what it means to be fully human. According to the pope, unions are "an indispensable element of social life."[9] They are impossible to ignore. Even if unions fail to make a difference in the immediate work place, the possibility of workers' joining together in association will affect society at large, the indirect employer.[10]

The strong emphasis on workers' right to organize has been central to Catholic social teaching. Unionism is the principle. A particular union that embodies that principle may be good or bad. Even a problematic or corrupt union, however, provides no excuse for rejecting the general principle of workers' right to unionize, no more than the many and obvious flaws in a particular church legitimizes rejecting all churches.

Unions and the Common Good

Fourth, unions and workers not in unions are responsible for promoting the common good in the relationship with management. In Catholic social teaching, unionism is not a form of class struggle. Unions have a responsibility to cooperate with management. Theirs is a struggle for the common good, not a struggle for the individual goods of workers unrelated to the common good. It cannot be egotistic. It must take account of the total socioeconomic justice needed. Basic community services must be safeguarded. Unions must not hold the whole of society hostage to their particular advancements. Rather, these advancements must always be seen in the perspective of the common good.

The Church as Model

There is one final point I want to highlight in the church's social teaching on unions and on human work. The church must be a model in its institutions of the social teaching. In 1971, the Synod of Bishops met and released the statement *Justice in the World*. In that statement they claimed that action on behalf of justice is central to proclaming the gospel. The institutions and the structures of our political and economic systems should reflect the gospel value of respect for human dignity, and the church must promote justice as part of its mission. The Synod then went on to observe:

> While the church is bound to give witness to justice, she recognizes that anyone who ventures to speak to people about justice must first be just in their eyes. Hence, we must undertake an examination of the modes of acting and of the possessions and lifestyle found within the church itself.[11]

Economic Justice for All emphasizes the same themes. The church must be a model of the justice it calls for,[12] even in the matter of unions.

> All church institutions must demonstrate this commitment to justice. All church institutions must also fully recognize the rights of employees to organize and bargain collectively with the institution through whatever association or organization they freely choose. In the light of new creative models of collaboration between labor and management described earlier in this letter, we challenge our church institutions to adopt new fruitful modes of cooperation. Although the church has its own nature and mission that must be respected and fostered, we are pleased that many who are not of our faith, but who share similar hopes and aspirations for the human family, work for us and with us in achieving this vision. In seeking greater justice in wages, we recognize the need to be alert particularly to the continuing discrimination against women throughout church and society, especially reflected in both the inequities of salaries between women and men and in the concentration of women in jobs at the lower end of the wage scale.[13]

The church would be justly accused of hypocrisy and scandal were any of its agencies to try to prevent the organization of unions by intimidation or coercion. Thus the new code of canon law insists that administrators in the church must observe meticulously the civil laws pertaining to labor and social policy according to church principles in the employment of workers. Clear policy should be established within all church agencies to ensure that workers' rights are respected.[14]

The U.S. bishops' *Health and Health Care* contains an even stronger statement on behalf of unions.

> An important and indispensible responsibility of employers in healthcare is the duty to deal justly with all employees. This involves not only just wages, fringe benefits and the like, but also the effective honoring of the desire of the employees "to be treated as free and responsible women and men able to participate in the decisions which affect their life and their future." This calls for the full recognition of the rights of employees to organize and bargain collectively with the institution through whatever association or organization they freely choose or through whatever other means seem appropriate without unjust pressures from their employers or from the already existing labor organizations.[15]

Guidelines

If we are to follow church teaching on labor, some guidelines would be helpful for putting the principles into action. The guidelines I am proposing here are suggested in the article "Ethical Guidelines for Religious Institutions Confronted by a Union" by Ed Marciniak.[16] They should be read within the overriding context of this discussion: the priority of healthcare ministry and the subordinate—although important—role of the healthcare industry model for understanding our work.

For Management

I want to suggest five basic guidelines for the *management* of healthcare institutions. First, reject paternalism. Administrators cannot look at employees as *only* employees. Second, reject all

148

vestiges of an antiunion mentality when the question of unionization arises. Unionization is central to Catholic social teaching. Third, Catholic health institutions must reject any third party influence that is blatantly antiunion or disrespectful of the church's social teaching. We cannot have on our premises any group that is blatantly antiunion any more than we can have a group that is openly proabortion. Fourth, avoid stereotypes. Do not let traditional ideas of "union types" as unreasonable or inflexible influence decision-making processes. Fifth, recognize that bargaining units for unions can also be a new resource for meeting some common problems. Labor-management relations need not be adversarial. We are all together in a ministry that is struggling to survive. We must forget the zero-sum notion of bargaining and concentrate on creative means to formulate policies, goals, and coresponsibility.[17]

For Unions

I also want to offer five guidelines for the *unions* which outline their responsibilities to healthcare ministry. First, respect the institution's nonprofit, service-oriented mission. The union is not bargaining with General Motors. Second, keep up-to-date on Catholic social teaching, especially the developments associated with the U.S. bishops pastoral on the economy. Third, reject the traditional hard-line approach. Unions must cooperate in the bargaining process. Fourth, avoid stereotypes of administrators as noncooperative and paternalistic. Finally, seek to be a resource for the whole community. It is important not to narrow the scope simply to isolated union interests.

For the Public

Here are five guidelines for the public at large. First, recognize the very difficult situation in which both healthcare institutions and unions find themselves. Unionization in the healthcare field is a new experience for both sides. Second, avoid stereotypes on either side, namely, seeing only good or only evil on one side. Third, hold both healthcare institutions and bargaining unions accountable to Catholic social teaching. Fourth, recognize that justice can be costly. Improved wages and better pensions for workers will probably add to medical expenses. Fifth, emphasize the wider content of the institution-union struggle, the societywide struggle to build more just structures that respect human dignity and promote human rights.

Challenge in the Vocation of Healthcare Employees

I believe that the issue of unionization within Catholic healthcare must ultimately be set within the context of the major challenges facing institutions as they move into the 1990s. The first and most obvious challenge is to keep the healthcare ministry model alive and functioning. There is a fast-growing group of healthcare institutions in this country that do not include ministry as a part of their mission statement or view it as a controlling factor in their decision making. These are the for-profit institutions. Roughly 15 percent of all healthcare institutions, including 80 percent of nursing care, are in the hands of for-profit corporations. Thus to keep ministry alive is a tremendous challenge and relates directly to the identity of Catholic healthcare.

A second challenge for Catholic institutions is the call to investigate alternatives in healthcare. Catholic institutions in their earlier days were precisely established to provide alternatives—reaching out to sectors of society that were ignored, offering services in the context of Christian vision, involving members of religious orders of women and men. Today, the alternatives in healthcare involve a whole host of approaches, very congruent with a ministry emphasis. These include healthcare education, prevention programs, holistic approaches, community-based services, spiritual healing, "high-touch/low-tech approaches," and so on. Catholic institutions can and should be pioneers in the alternatives approach.[18]

Third, Catholic healthcare must creatively implement the basic option for the poor. As I have emphasized elsewhere,[19] the option for the poor should not be implemented in a reductionist fashion, simply as providing services for those who cannot pay fees. As important as this is, the option for the poor requires much more by way of corporate stances. These stances include hiring and promotion policies, purchasing practices, and investment practices. The institution's overall corporate stance within the local community must be evaluated in terms of its political impact (e.g., regarding support of health insurance programs), the

150

economic consequences of its decisions (e.g., land-use decisions), and the cultural meaning of its operations (e.g., the diversity of its boards). All these elements have significant bearing at the institution's option for the poor.

These three challenges—the ministry model, alternatives, and the option for the poor—confront all participants in Catholic healthcare: management, unions, and nonunion employees. How they respond will depend in a fundamental way upon how they look at their work.

I have been helped to understand different perspectives on work by a distinction recently made by Robert Bellah and his associates in their important study, *Habits of the Heart.*[20] In their analysis of the tension in the United States between community and individualism, they suggest that we tend to view work in three different ways: (1) as a *job*, something that must be done so that I can do something else; (2) as a *career*, something I do for upward mobility, to achieve, to gain recognition, and perquisites; and (3) as a *vocation*, something I feel called to, to be part of something much larger, to be part of the transformation of our society.

This distinction certainly has relevance to the very viability of Catholic healthcare ministry in our country today. If all who work in it—whether management or labor, whether in a union or not—see their work as a vocation and struggle to see that their sense of vocation shapes all significant decisions, Catholic healthcare has a much more promising future. In that context, the issue of unionization changes character. The local unions can be seen as partners in ministry with sponsors, managers, and other workers. The security, strength, and resources they provide for their members become resources in service of the ministry and vocation of healthcare. That is the vision that Catholic social teaching holds up before us, the reality it calls us to create.

Footnotes
  1. This chapter is a revision of an address given by Peter Henriot, SJ, at the Catholic Hospital Administrative Personnel Program, Sept. 2, 1985.
  2. Vatican Council II, *Pastoral Constitution on the Church in the Modern World,* #1 in Walter M. Abbott, SJ, *The Documents of Vatican II,* America Press, New York, 1966, pp. 199-200.
  3. For more on these issues, see Chapter 2, "Catholic Healthcare: Competing and Complementary Models," and Chapter 5, "Service of the Poor: The Foundation of Judeo-Christian Response."

4. For a fuller discussion of several of these points, see Chapter 2, "Catholic Healthcare: Competing and Complementary Models."

5. Charles Craypo, PhD, and Rev. Patrick J. Sullivan, CSC, PhD, "Unions and Catholic Health Care Facilities," *Issues in the Labor Management Dialogue: Church Perspectives*, Adam J. Maida, ed., The Catholic Health Association of the United States, St. Louis, 1982, pp. 14-46.

6. Peter J. Henriot, Edward P. DeBerri, and Michael J. Schultheis, *Catholic Social Teaching: Our Best Kept Secret* Center of Concern/Orbis, Maryknoll, NY, 1988.

7. Pope John Paul II, *On Human Work, Origins*, vol. 11, no. 15, Sept. 244, 1981, pp. 225-244.

8. *Economic Justice for All: Pastoral Letter on Catholic Social Teaching and the U.S. Economy*, National Conference of Catholic Bishops, U.S. Catholic Conference, Washington, DC 1986, #136.

9. *On Human Work*, p. 239.

10. Pope John Paul distinguishes between the direct employer and the indirect employer. The direct employer is the person or the institution providing the job. The indirect employer is the wider society, which conditions and shapes the situation within which work goes on. The government, public institutions, other businesses, households, and consumers are all "indirect employers" of workers. See *On Human Work*, no. 17, p. 237.

11. *Justice in the World*, p. 40.

12. *Economic Justice for All: Pastoral Letter on Catholic Social Teaching and the U.S. Economy*, #326, #347.

13. *Economic Justice for All: Pastoral Letter on Catholic Social Teaching and the U.S. Economy*, #353. The first sentence of this quotation is a reference to the bishops' earlier pastoral letter, National Conference of Catholic Bishops, U.S. Catholic Conference, 1982, #50.

14. Canon Law #1286, section 1.

15. *Health and Health Care*, National Conference of Catholic Bishops, *Origins*, Vol. 11, No. 25, Dec. 3, 1981. The quotation within the quotation is from the Address of Pope John Paul II at Monterey, Mexico, Jan. 31, 1979.

16. See Ed Marciniak, "Ethical Guidelines for a Religious Institutions Confronted by a Union," *Social Thought*, Spring 1984, vol. X, no. 2.

17. For more on this, see Chapter 8, "The Call For a Prophetic Healthcare System."

18. See Chapter 1, "Building a Healthy Society: A Catholic Challenge of the Future."

19. See Chapter 5, "Service of the Poor: The Foundation of Judeo-Christian Response."

20. Robert N. Bellah, et al., *Habits of the Heart: Individualism and Commitment in American Society*, University of California Press, Berkeley, 1985.

Reflection Questions

1. This chapter examines church social teachings that provide the foundation for and give expression to workers' right to unionize. It examines two basic religious principles: the primacy of labor over capital, and the right of the worker to participate in the economic decisions that affect her or his life. The chapter maintains that the issue of unionization is not just one of many issues but is a central issue that will determine whether Catholic healthcare continues to offer viable ministry.

   • Do you agree with the importance the chapter places on this issue? Why or why not?

2. The chapter outlines some key elements of Catholic social teaching and explores their implications for healthcare ministry.

   • What are the five major teachings extracted from *On the Condition of Labor (Rerum Novarum)* and the Bishops' pastoral on the economy? How does your institution measure up in relation to them?

   • Can you see any common thread among the sets of guidelines outlined for management, employees, and the public at large? What are they?

   • In your experience, are the business aspects of healthcare positioned to serve the ministry?

   • How would an understanding of one's vocation in healthcare influence the decisions of healthcare workers?

3. This chapter discusses the concept of work at great length. It reiterates Pope John Paul II's views that work is the key element that allows life to become more human and that making life more human is the social question of our times. It uses Robert Bellah's differentiation of job, career, and vocation to put in relief the impact of considering work as a vocation.

   • Do you think these views and their implications are understood and accepted by most people in our culture? Why or why not?

   • Do you think these views operate in the marketplace? Why or why not?

   • How might they be introduced and operationalized in your institution(s)?

   • If this were done, what differences might be expected in social spheres?

· 10 ·

Generating a Truly *Catholic* Response In Difficult Times[1]

James E. Hug, SJ

In Chapter 4, I described the struggles facing Catholic healthcare institutions today as a textbook case of the stresses inherent in the relationship between Christian social values and a capitalist market economy.[2] During the late 1960s and through the 1970s Catholic healthcare had the financial breathing space to begin developing an institutional identity embodying Catholic social vision and principles. In the 1980s, its relatively protected economic environment was invaded and it is now being pushed into stiffer and stiffer market competition. Can Catholic healthcare institutions survive this environmental shift with their Catholic social identity intact?

I hope—and assume—that it is possible for Catholic healthcare to work within the U.S. economic system with Christian social integrity. That same hope is reflected in the U.S. bishops' pastoral letter on Catholic social teaching and the U.S. economy when it suggests that business management can be seen as a Christian *vocation* when it is carried out in service of the larger public good and not simply the corporation's private good.[3]

But is that a realistic hope? I am afraid the data are increasingly foreboding. Market forces are, without a doubt, excluding the medically indigent from adequate healthcare and are pushing us toward a two-tiered or multitiered healthcare system.[4] The pressure to cut costs puts a premium on keeping wages as low as possible. There seems to be a serious competitive disadvantage in respecting the long-standing Catholic moral commit-ment to labor's right to organize.[5]

In addition, the search for markets necessarily encourages programs that respond to the needs of those segments of the population able to pay for them. *The effective language of the market is money: the crisis of those without it cannot be heard in the marketplace.* Highly competitive markets subtly generate *programming* and *institutional development* geared toward the upper strata of the economy.

Market pressures in healthcare can also generate destruc-tive forms of competition. Recently five Washington, DC hospitals (including a major Catholic hospital) applied for permission to perform heart transplants despite the fact that transplant programs in Baltimore, MD, and Richmond, VA, are already more than adequate to meet the region's transplant needs for years to come. Institutional prestige increases market share. In this case, compe-tition for that prestige seems to have blotted out consideration of regional medical need and public welfare. These institutions had not yet heard or understood the call of the economic pastoral to explore new forms of regional collaboration for the sake of the common good.[6]

On a somewhat different scale, I have heard Catholic Charities directors complaining of Catholic hospitals undercutting some of their health programs in the scramble for lucrative new markets to shore up the struggling institutions. Competition can be valuable, but not when it wastes resources and undercuts the sense of community solidarity in mission that we should be nurturing within the church community.

It is increasingly clear that what we face is not just a challenge to become better business managers. The market system today in the United States does not share some of our most impor-tant Catholic social values. And it presses us to conform to its values—or die. The effort to maintain Catholic values in today's business environment demands more than a "balancing act." It demands a prophetic challenge to the system's structures.

The entrance of Catholic healthcare into the national policy debates in recent years is an encouraging sign that it is taking its responsibility to prophetic leadership seriously. But I am afraid that it remains a slim ray of hope in a dismal picture. At a 1986 conference, "The Healthcare Gap and How to Bridge It,"[7] the congressional speakers repeatedly encouraged the healthcare community to continue advocating for the poor. That was their first sentence. Their second sentence warned that little progress will be possible for the foreseeable future. The massive federal deficit and the Gramm-Rudman-Hollings Balanced Budget Act have combined to create a potentially lethal depressant for the next few generations' healthcare concerns. The picture they sketched has grown even grimmer in recent months as the federal government struggles to face the implications of the stock market crash of Oct. 19, 1987.

I do not want to underestimate Catholic healthcare ability to generate broad and effective national coalitions to advocate care for the poor and the rebuilding of a single-tiered healthcare system serving everyone in the nation equitably. Nor do I want to overlook its great creativity in generating and nurturing new approaches to healthcare within the constraints of the current socioeconomic context. On the contrary, I want to encourage both wholeheartedly. They are essential to Catholic managerial integrity. On the other hand, I do not want to be naive about the possibilities for fidelity to Catholic social imperatives as the "marketizing" of U.S. healthcare continues.

Deepening the Challenge

That is a sketch of the situation as I see it reflected in the life and literature of U.S. Catholic healthcare today. It is a difficult and uneasy situation, one that is only too familiar to people working in the field. I am still not satisfied, however, that this sketch puts the elements of the picture in proper perspective. I am afraid that we have only begun to probe the depths and dimensions of the challenge before us, of the prophetic vocation being offered us in the signs of our times.

My first observation is that the debate over healthcare for the poor and medically indigent is being carried on completely within a national horizon. The literature, the discussions, and the legislative advocacy all focus exclusively on providing for the medical needs of the U.S. poor. And yet the *Catholic* vision of the common good is *universal*. If the right to adequate healthcare is a basic human right—as official Catholic teaching and Catholic healthcare personnel have argued for many years now—then it is a right of all human beings no matter what their national origin or geographic location. Human rights are grounded, as the U.S. pastoral on the economy puts it, in "an inalienable dignity that stamps human existence prior to any division into races or nations and prior to human labor and human achievement (Gen.4-11)."[8]

I was in El Salvador during Holy Week in 1986, and I spent a good deal of time in some of the refugee camps set up by the church to shelter those displaced from their land by the war. In one camp, two U.S. women religious had set up a small clinic. I saw the skimpy collection of aspirin, Maalox, gauze pads, and other minimal medications they had to treat everything from scraped knees to shrapnel wounds, ulcers and sleeplessness to diarrhea, malnutrition, malaria, tetanus, typhoid, and tuberculosis. One of the women said, "We don't need an electron microscope. We just need the most basic microscope to do simple blood tests!" Then she added almost immediately, "But I was a hospital adminis-trator in the States, and I know that the shipping costs can be prohibitive."

Many people in U.S. Catholic healthcare institutions know people in situations like that. They may be members of the same religious communities who are trying to respond to the over-whelming needs found in Third World barrios and rural villages. Perhaps they worked with us in this country before they went there. Through them the suffering and needs of the world's poor can become very real and personal. The basic right of these poor to healthcare makes a claim on us. It is a prophetic challenge that cannot make itself heard above the growing noise of the national marketplace. It is a call echoed in the words of the economic pastoral:

> From the Patristic period to the present, the church
> has affirmed that misuse of the world's resources or
> appropriation of them by a minority of the world's
> population betrays the gift of creation since "whatever
> belongs to God belongs to all."[9]

Response to their need is not simply a government responsibility. It falls on all of us, personally and corporately. They are our brothers, sisters, and neighbors more fundamentally than they are foreigners or enemies.

But what good does this type of reflection do? It probably alienates more people than it inspires. When people in Catholic healthcare are feeling beleaguered by the healthcare situation in the United States, the suggestion that they should also be thinking somehow about the massive healthcare needs of the world's poor sounds outrageous. How can we involve ourselves in global issues when we cannot devote ourselves to the needs of our own poor without facing bankruptcy?

The fact is, we are all already deeply immersed in global issues. The economic constraints currently being imposed and the rising number of medically indigent knocking at the doors of healthcare institutions are in significant part domestic manifestations of global economic shifts. The technological developments that have transformed modern medicine and sent its costs skyrocketing have also transformed industry. Automation has replaced millions of jobs. Advances in communications and transportation, combining with the competitive pressures of the market system, have enabled (and, in some instances, forced) the flight of industry from the United States to the cheap labor markets and unregulated environments of the Third World.

In many of those environments, uncontrolled industrial pollution is generating a flood of diseases that the local healthcare systems cannot handle. Transnational corporate policies and development programs devised in the industrialized world contribute to the growing gap between wealthy and poor nations.

The global industrial shift toward the Third World is not "trickling down" to alleviate deprivation of the poor or the debt of their nations. These are worsening in most places, and global health suffers as a consequence.

Meanwhile at home, the loss of employment, the poverty, and the decay of local communities due to capital flight are generating a variety of stress-related health problems in the mushrooming medically indigent population. Loss of employment generally means loss of insurance for the working person and her or his dependents. Our culture has long linked personal worth and productivity, and so it is not surprising that healthcare insurance was first provided through the workplace—or that the workplace is still the major source of insurance protection for most Americans under the age of 65.

At the same time, massive military spending is con-suming resources—financial, industrial and human—that could be used to rebuild the U.S. economy and meet the needs of those who bear the greatest part of the burden imposed by this global economic transition. The nuclear threat grows by the day, threatening the world's population with insoluble health problems that the Chernobyl tragedy only begins to hint at. The United States is watching its smokestack industries being exiled to the Third World and more and more of its middle class slipping toward poverty. The trade balance worsens. A "deficit mentality" reigns, and social programs for the poor and medically indigent wither or are aborted before they see the light of day. The mood of our country is currently protectionist, nationalistic, and militaristic.

The Economic Pastoral

This is the context in which the U.S. bishops encourage us to resist our nationalistic and protectionist instincts. They ask us to meditate on the creation narratives, remembering that *all* people reflect God's image and are equally God's chosen and loved. We are called to a covenant aimed at nurturing community with *all*, community that is characterized by mutual respect, collabora-tion, and special care for the poor.[10]

The human tendency to pull back and defend ourselves and our way of living must be faced and challenged. The Gospel imperative of universal love sometimes calls us to remain open, with arms outstretched to our sisters and brothers, even when that is crucifying. If the management imperative of institutional survival becomes absolute, we are living heresy. Survival was clearly not an absolute value for Jesus. He chose to accept death rather than be unfaithful to his mission. Faithful followers of Jesus, then, obviously cannot consider survival—whether personal or institutional—essential to the mission.

Some Implications

Where do these considerations take us? What do they imply for the daily problems of keeping healthcare institutions and systems afloat and actively committed to the Catholic mission of healing today? I will not pretend to have the answers to these questions, but I do have a few suggestions that arise in part from work already begun.

First, to make sure that our Gospel imperatives govern our response to business imperatives, we must all work to maintain a *perspective* and an *active concern* that are *global* as well as national, regional, and local. That perspective and concern will help those involved in Catholic healthcare arrive at a more realistic sense of their identity. They will see it in comparison with other national healthcare systems and conditions. To state it somewhat provocatively, it will enable them to evaluate their investment of money, energies, and resources in maintaining a qualified and committed Catholic presence in a national healthcare system that

- Is technologically driven
- Produces great breakthroughs in medical knowledge and skill
- Is in service of a work ethic in which personal value is still largely associated with productivity
- Demands massive resources and gradually orients them to serve fewer and wealthier people
- Seemingly responds to a cultural fear of death by helping those with the resources to afford it to hold off death at almost any cost
- Is gradually losing its sensitivity to the basic health needs of the poor nationally and is almost totally oblivious of health needs of the global poor
- Is weak in its commitment to primary and preventive healthcare.

The call to take a global perspective is not the only implication of the *Catholic* dimension of our identity. Catholic healthcare workers are members of one of the largest transnational corporate networks on earth. There is coordinated Catholic institutional presence in every part of the world. Those associated with religious communities who have missionaries in other parts of the world may think of themselves as belonging to independently owned "transnational subsidiaries."

Most of these transnational institutional links—these bridges to the global poor—have not yet been developed in ways that could further the church's corporate healing mission. During the 1960s many U.S. dioceses developed twinning relationships with Latin American dioceses; recently U.S. Jesuits have been exploring the possibility of greater resource sharing with Central American Jesuit institutions. Perhaps it is time for U.S. Catholic healthcare systems and institutions to develop effective trans-national links to extend Christ's healing touch. The church structures are there to help bridge the gap and form this type of relationship.[11]

In recent decades, communities with institutional relationships into the Third World have come to recognize that they are not uni-directional. The poor of the earth have a great deal to teach the so-called developed nations about human life and Christian mission. They can, for example, help us to keep our management decisions in a more realistic Gospel context. When we think of those working in healthcare in the Third World not so much as heroic individuals, missionaries working in terrible conditions of hardship, but more as our sisters and brothers, colleagues in our corporate healing ministry whose responsibilities and struggles are in some way our responsibilities and struggles too, then our operational decisions and priorities take on a different significance. The decision to purchase an electron microscope or to establish a heart transplant unit must be weighed not simply in the light of an individual hospital's resources, needs, desires, and competitive status, but also in relationship to the lack of any microscope for basic blood tests or the lack of basic heart medications in other parts of our corporate healing mission.

It is not yet clear what practical results might flow from this shift in perspective. In some cases it could mean reorientation of an institution's programming to give priority to primary and preventive healthcare in the United States and greater sharing of resources with sister/brother institutions in the Third World. Such a shift would probably require significant educational efforts with trustees, staff, and the general public to explain the values involved and to highlight the importance of primary healthcare. That is an important and needed form of evangelization for U.S. culture.

In other cases this shift in perspective might involve creative personnel exchange programs and equipment sharing. Personal involvement in carrying out the healing mission in Third World conditions is a powerful experience that is worth sharing as broadly as possible. Some schools and healthcare institutions are already engaged in this type of activity, sending teams on rotation to different parts of the world where institutional links have been established. In some cases this shift in perspective may involve finding ways to make sophisticated diagnostic resources available to the poor of the world through relatively inexpensive satellite hookups with Third World clinics. And in practically all cases, it will mean broadening the agenda of legislative advocacy to accommodate this wider conception of the Catholic healing mission.

Conclusion

I offer these few suggestions in the hope that they will stimulate imaginations and encourage the sharing and exploration of similar ideas and experiences. I believe we must expand our horizons to maintain and develop our mission's catholicity in today's world. I recognize that first steps in the directions I have suggested will be cautious and tentative. Global problems, too, are only solved small step by small step. I recognize as well that these small steps will generate further hard decisions in the future. But I also believe that these directions promise ways of constructively redirecting energies and resources currently in danger of being wasted in unnecessary, destructive competition here at home.

It is becoming increasingly clear that the current global economic transition generating the current pressures in Catholic healthcare institutions and systems is in part a prophetic call from God to conversion from the worst facets of our market economy.

For us, it represents an invitation to help transform attitudes, institutional structures, and systems that
- Overtechnologize healthcare and are governed by technological imperatives
- Emerge from and embody our cultural fear of death
- Serve our cultural tendency to identify human worth with productivity
- Express our individualism and nationalism
- Exclude from our concern too many of the poor, domestically and globally

My point is: The right balance of Catholic and management imperatives at this time in history in this nation must not be narrowed to "How can we compete and survive and still provide (our share of) care for the nation's poor and medically indigent?" We face much more basic questions. We should be asking: "Can we continue to contribute to the development of the

U.S. healthcare system in the current global context with integrity as Catholic Christians guided by the imperative of universal love?"

And if we can answer "yes" to that, we must ask:

- How do we want to try to guide and shape its development?
- How can we help to reverse the national trend toward dominance of healthcare by market forces that cater preferentially to those with money?
- How can we help to guarantee that healthcare can remain mission driven rather than becoming market driven?
- How can we help to heal our cultural diseases that overvalue productivity and identify it too closely with human worth, that exaggerate the evil of death, and that magnify the redemptive possibilities of technology?
- How can we foster international perspectives for more effective transnational healing to restore wholeness, *shalom,* peace to our world?

To return to the point I began with, I still consider Catholic healthcare a crucial test case for clarifying the relationship between Catholic social values and the U.S. economic system. The issues and challenges seem more complex by the day. Whatever successes Catholic healthcare achieves will be important models for institutions that share our values in all sectors of the economy. They will also be redemptive, healing influences—special sacraments of healing in a world that badly needs this Catholic healing touch.

Footnotes

1. This chapter is a revision of an address by James E. Hug, SJ, given at the 71st Annual Catholic Health Assembly.
2. See Chapter 4, "Capitalism and Christian Values: A Process for Discernment."
3. *Economic Justic for All: Pastoral Letter on Catholic Social Teaching and the U.S. Economy,* National Conference of Catholic Bishops, U.S. Catholic Conference, Washington, DC, 1986, #115, see also #108-114.
4. *No Room in the Marketplace: The Health Care of the Poor,* The Catholic Health Association, St. Louis, 1986, pp. 1-13.
5. For a discussion of the positive potential of unions for healthcare institutions in the current crisis, see Chapter 8, "The Call for a Prophetic Healthcare System."
6. *Economic Justice for All: Pastoral Letter on Catholic Social Teaching and the U.S. Economy,* Chapter 4, "A New American Experiment: Partnership for the Common Good."
7. *Who Cares? The Health Care Gap and How to Bridge It,* Women's Research and Education Institute, Washington, DC, 1987.

8. *Economic Justice for All: Pastoral Letter on Catholic Social Teaching and the U.S. Economy,* #32.
9. *Economic Justice for All: Pastoral Letter on Catholic Social Teaching and the U.S. Economy,* #34.
10. *Economic Justice for All: Pastoral Letter on Catholic Social Teaching and the U.S. Economy,* #267-270, pp. 31-40.
11. Indeed, some work along these lines is already going on. A survey of transnational efforts is available from the Catholic Health Association in a paper by Elizabeth McMillan (as yet unpublished at the time of this writing).

Reflection Questions

1. The chapter opens with a bleak narrative of the economic realities of our day and cautions us not to be naive about the possibilities for fidelity to Catholic social imperatives as the "marketizing" of U.S. healthcare continues.
   - Can Catholic institutions survive this environmental shift with their Catholic social identity intact? What is your response? Explain.

2. The chapter suggests that one way of expressing the Catholic identity is to reorient systems, giving priority to services that are primary and preventive, and to share these services throughout the world.
   - Would you agree to this focus? Why or why not?
   - What "small tentative steps" would you suggest to begin to educate Catholic healthcare providers to the desirability of moving in this direction?
   - What services would you identify as preventive and primary?

3. In the face of the problems cited above, our human tendency to pull back and to defend ourselves and our way of living must be challenged. The bishops urge us to resist our nationalistic and protectionistic instincts and to take enormous risks to propose Catholic values.
   - Can a disproportionate consumption of healthcare resources by the United States be justified in the light of global poverty and need? Explain.
   - How can we afford to involve ourselves in global issues when we cannot care for the needs of our own poor without facing bankruptcy?

4. Religious congregations of men and women have a singular opportunity to cut across national boundaries and develop effective transnational links to extend Christ's healing touch throughout the entire world.
   - How can we work more effectively to develop and maintain a perspective and an active concern that is global as well as national, regional, and local.

5. The imperative to universal love calls us to probe to the heart of the problems besetting us today. We seem to have a prophetic call from God to depart from the status quo and to open ourselves to conversion from the worst facets of our present market economy.

   • What is your response to the questions raised at the end of this chapter?

· 11 ·

Church Influence in the Economics of Healthcare: Implications of
Economic Justice for All: Pastoral Letter on Catholic Social Teaching and the U.S. Economy[1]

James E. Hug, SJ

Can the church influence the economics of healthcare in the United States? That question cannot be isolated from the larger issue of the U.S. role in the global economy. Healthcare economics cannot be understood independently of national and international economies and the cultural forces that shape and support them.

As the economic pastoral itself points out, one of the central signs of our times (i.e., one of the central carriers of God's revelation to us today)[2] is the growing interdependence of all elements of the global economy and the role of the United States in it.[3] One clear implication of this is that the future of healthcare economics will only be understood adequately if it is recognized to be tied to the future of national and global economies.

But if healthcare economics is tied to national and global economics, so too is the very foundation of healthcare economics: people's *health*. Poverty and unemployment not only create a crisis for healthcare reimbursement, they also generate a variety of health problems that compound the reimbursement issues, problems ranging from stress-related diseases and increased domestic violence to substance abuse and rising rates of infant mortality.[4] Poverty brings malnourishment, which breeds diminished mental and physical capacities. It thereby guarantees greater social problems and fewer human resources to deal with them in the future. Any healthcare today that aspires to cure many of the diseases it encounters must include vigorous assaults on unemployment and poverty—local, regional, national, and international. Such assaults are as integral to adequate healthcare in our world as the ongoing research into the causes of cancer or acquired immune deficiency syndrome (AIDS).

The point of these introductory comments, then, is that it is necessary to look at the full range of the economic pastoral's concerns if we want to discover its implications for healthcare economics and its potential influence on them.

In trying to do that, I will organize my reflections under three headings:

1. The church's potential influence on healthcare economics through this pastoral letter is greatly strengthened by the *process* through which it was formulated.
2. Its influence rests on its analysis of the economic and cultural forces at work among us and its interpretation of them in the light of Christian faith and tradition.
3. The church's influence rests on its integrity in modeling the justice it calls for.

The Influence of the Process

In developing the economic pastoral, the U.S. Catholic bishops used a process designed to pool the best resources available and to make it as much as possible a document of the whole church community. A drafting committee began with several years of study and more than 20 hearings across the country involving experts in economics, politics, theology, ethics, and related disciplines. In November 1984 they published a first draft of the proposed letter and asked for responses from anyone who wished. The 10,000-plus pages of response they received shaped the second draft, which was published a year later. The same procedure of national debate led to a third draft in the summer of 1986. That draft was further amended and finally passed by the bishops' conference in November 1986.

The open, participative process strengthened the document considerably by drawing on the vast resources of the whole Catholic community. This is not simply the bishops' pastoral letter. It is the church's pastoral letter coordinated, formulated, and published by the bishops. For that reason, a number of blanket criticisms of the letter arising from the complaint that the bishops are not economists and do not know what they are talking about miss the point. In this letter, as in the peace pastoral, community participation and expertise—including some of the best economists and social scientists available—directly shaped Catholic teaching.

This participative process was consciously chosen to operationalize the Second Vatican Council's theological insight that the church is the People of God. It should not be identified with the hierarchy of pope, bishops, and clergy. In fostering the notion that all of us are the church and engaging us in the formation of Catholic social teaching, the bishops were enhancing the church's influence on economic issues (including healthcare issues) in other ways as well. They were challenging us, for example, to see economic issues as moral and religious issues. This contradicts the assignment of religion to private life, which is one of the legacies of the Enlightenment and one of our culture's often unquestioned assumptions. It is an assumption that must be corrected if the church is to influence healthcare economics. The pastoral states it strongly:

> Explicit reflection on the ethical content of economic choices and policies must become an integral part of the way Christians relate religious belief to the realities of everyday life. In this way, the "split between the faith which many profess and their daily lives," which Vatican II counted among the more serious errors of the modern age, will begin to be bridged.[5]

As the church community grows in awareness of the religious and moral significance of economic decisions, policies, and structures, an important and influential constituency for social change will form.

Second, dialogue between the bishops and the community and the bishops' respect for the contributions of all strengthened and rebuilt the church's community life. The bishops had developed a process to prepare us for more active participation in reshaping national economic and cultural life. When people are enabled to participate meaningfully in shaping their community's self-understanding, decisions, and activities, they gain self-respect and become more active citizens, assuming more responsibility for the common good.[6]

Third, this understanding of church implies—to paraphrase Pogo—that "we have met the church's influence in healthcare economics, and it is us." As members of God's people, leaders in church-related healthcare institutions are principal carriers of the church's influence in this arena. They do not stand alone in that role. They are only "the pope and bishops" of healthcare institutions and systems. To generate and guide the church's immediate direct influence in healthcare economics, they must draw on the entire community's resources. They must invite and nurture the active participation of all those who work in the system, those who are served through it, and those who are affected by it in developing their orientation and policies for dealing with the difficult economic realities they face.

In this context, the commitment to collaboration is extremely significant. It must not simply be collaboration with leaders in other institutions or systems. It must permeate institutions and systems. That is more difficult, as we all know, than using the rhetoric of collaboration and participation rather than its reality. But once truly participative structures operate, they will generate thousands of bearers of the church's influence, bringing their talents to help transform our socioeconomic context.

The Influence of Analysis and Interpretation

My second general point is that the church's influence on healthcare economics through this pastoral will rest on the letter's analysis of the economic and cultural forces at work today and its interpretation of them in the light of Christian faith and tradition.

Economic Analysis

The analysis has two facets: *economic* and *cultural*. The economic analysis highlights the new mobility of capital and technology that has made global production and trade possible. In many industries, wages have become the main variable in the cost of production. This, of course, gives significant advantage to those who produce their products in the nations of the Third World where the standard of living and the cost of labor are very low: As the letter states,

> Overseas competitors with the same technology but with wage rates as low as one-tenth of ours put enormous pressure on U.S. firms to cut wages, relocate abroad, or close.[7]

U.S. industry has been seriously hurt, and the list of casualties continues to grow: textiles, clothing, shoes, steel, automobiles, audio and video equipment, microchips, computers, and peripherals. Recently a columnist described in *The New York Times* waking up to discover that 85 percent of the things in his apartment came from Japan. Japan produced his alarm clock, bicycle, camera, fan, guitar, hair dryer, iron, humidifier, microwave oven, razor, stereo, pencil sharpener, telephone, tennis racket, toaster oven, Walkman, and television. America, he decided, contributed his country and western albums, books, and food.[8] He is probably wrong about the food, however, since the United States imports a great deal of food.

Even so, his fantasy contains a great deal of truth. Hundreds of thousands of jobs in industrial production have been lost. More than 90 percent of the jobs created to replace them since the early 1970s have been in the service sector. Most of those pay poorly: 95 percent of the service sector jobs created in the last year, for example, are in the lowest paying categories—near or below the poverty level.[9] And it has become commonplace in the industry that remains to use the threat of plant closings to force acceptance of pay cuts and other concessions from workers—whether union members or not.

In general, the middle class continues to suffer erosion. The gap between wealthy and poor is growing, both nationally and globally. The only ways for the United States to increase its productivity and global competitiveness would appear to be through cutting wages and benefits and increasing mechanization or robotization. Neither would improve the economic outlook for the majority of U.S. citizens or their healthcare providers. Both would help make the rich richer and the poor poorer.

The fact that this situation is the result of technological breakthroughs and relatively stable international socioeconomic realities indicates this problem's structural nature. It will not be solved by replacing a few greedy personnel with more generous ones. We are in the midst of a major global economic transition whose significance, in my judgment, rivals that of the Industrial Revolution.

This analysis suggests two important implications for healthcare economics. First, we are not dealing with a short-term problem. It is a structural adjustment of the world economy. Even if we see some upturn in the U.S. economy, it is hard to see how it would significantly reduce unemployment, create the kind of jobs that would carry adequate healthcare benefits, or generate the political will to provide more federal and state funds to cover healthcare costs for the indigent. Second, if economic developments continue consolidating the national wealth in the hands of fewer people, the pressures on healthcare deliverers to serve their needs and desires will increase. Providers of healthcare will be pressured to provide more upscale services to those who can afford them—and forced to watch their effective commitment to healthcare for the poor eroded.

Cultural Analysis

The cultural analysis offered by the pastoral is also quite significant. It arises from diagnostic reflection upon the growing array of economic problems challenging us. The diagnosis is this: our mushrooming economic problems are

> Symptoms of more fundamental currents shaping U.S. economic life today: the struggle to find meaning and value in human work, efforts to support individual freedom in the context of renewed social cooperation, the urgent need to create equitable forms of global interdependence in a world now marked by extreme inequality. These deeper currents are cultural and moral in content. They show that the long-range challenges facing the nation call for sustained reflection on the values that guide economic choices and are embodied in economic institutions.[10]

The cultural values contributing to our decaying economic situation have roots in the Enlightenment and the Industrial Revolution. Specialization and the division of labor, although they have produced great advances in many sectors of our society (including medicine), have given us a population trained to focus more and more on less and less. The price of entering the economy is the ability to define oneself and one's work narrowly enough to find a niche in the marketplace.

The costs of our national commitment to specialization and the division of labor are not often accounted. For one thing, they generate social passivity. We are aware that we do not know much beyond our narrow realm of work and are intimidated by the "experts." Medical practitioners have exploited this situation for years. Some healthcare systems are now insisting that individuals assume primary responsibility for their own health. They present themselves as assistants to these individuals in the active promotion and facilitation of healing.[11] This is a reversal of current general expectations, however. Although a positive development, it will require long, slow, gentle education for both patients and medical personnel to overcome patients' passivity.

The costs of specialization and the division of labor also include a loss of a sense of the whole, of how things work together. Those who focus too long and hard at close-range details lose the ability to see the larger world. As people lose their sense of the whole, they naturally focus more on personal goals and private interests.[12] They can only see clearly what is within their shortened range of focus. The long-term effect of these phenomena is social fragmentation, heightened individualism, the loss of a common moral vision, and the disappearance of commitment to the common good. We argue, "What I have is mine. I earned it. I can do anything I want with it. If others don't have it, it's their own fault. They didn't work hard enough; they didn't compete hard enough."

These are some of the values that enable corporations pursuing increased profits to close and move profitable plants without any concern for the impact on the workers or the local communities. These are some of the values that encourage upper management in major corporations and industries to take millions of dollars in bonuses while laying off thousands of workers.[13] These are some of the values that impel corporations to dump their wastes

173

into the environment without any sense of responsibility for ecological damage or community health problems. These are some of the values that support the driving of healthcare into the market-place and the unwillingness to finance care for the medically indigent.

As should be painfully clear, these cultural values are serious health hazards. Unless they are changed, there seems to be little realistic hope of significant improvement in the current economic situation of the nation—and, therefore, in the current economic situation of healthcare.

Theological Interpretation

The pastoral's economic and cultural analyses enable us to understand our current situation a bit more clearly, but its *theological interpretation* of the situation provides the key to evaluating it and suggesting directions of response. To ground its theological reflection, the letter turns to the period of Israel's history known in the Jewish-Christian scriptures as the Babylonian Exile.[14] The suggestion implicit in this starting point is striking. It is this: Israel's experience in being exiled to Babylon is enough like our experience in the United States now that what God taught them through that experience is what God is trying to teach us now.

Why is our current experience like the Exile? Well, we have not been conquered militarily and taken as prisoners or slaves to a foreign land, but our economic supremacy has been overcome. We are no longer Number One. We are, in fact, the largest debtor nation in the world. And we are watching our jobs exiled by the hundreds of thousands. Small communities all across the nation are collapsing as their resources of wealth and talent are siphoned off. We speak of working harder to increase productivity and competitiveness; but as we have seen, the picture remains grim on those fronts. We are struggling as a nation with the loss of our global economic dominance—and with it the loss of our sense of identity as God's chosen nation, the beacon on the hill heralding the superiority of freedom, the bearers and defenders of religious and democratic values for the world. This is the same type of profound national identity crisis that the Babylonian Exile triggered for Israel.[15]

Through that experience, they learned some important lessons from God that the pastoral suggests as appropriate for us in our situation. They learned the profound dignity of *every* human being as God's child, created in God's own image. That sacred dignity is universal. It is more fundamental than nationality, race, gender, or accomplishment. It is the birthright of every man, woman, and child on this globe. They learned, too, that God gave the gifts of creation to provide for each person's needs. Everyone has an equal claim before God on the resources of the universe. It is a crime against God when some people hoard them while others lack for basic needs.

They also recalled the guidance for full and peaceful living that God had given them in the Covenant at Mount Sinai. They were to show love and respect for all people, but especially for the poor. They had not been faithful to that guidance; they had ignored the prophet's warnings. They realized that the Exile was the bitter medicine necessary to heal the community diseased by their national infidelity. The God who had liberated them from slavery in Egypt enslaved them in Babylon for the sake of their deeper liberation.

The same themes are present in Jesus' life and teaching.[16] He placed himself with the poor, faithful to his vocation to bring God's good news to them. He told parables showing the wealthy who hoard their riches without concern for the community to be fools in God's eyes and liable to the judgment and punishment handed out to Dives.[17] He called for our lives to be rooted in the compassion of the Good Samaritan. And in his story of the Last Judgment, he identified himself with the poor and needy of the world. As the pastoral puts it:

> The shock comes when [the cursed] find that in
> neglecting the poor, the outcast, and the oppressed,
> they were rejecting Jesus himself . . . . [T]o reject them
> is to reject God made manifest in history.[18]

Christian reflection through the centuries has thrown some further helpful light on these basic notions.[19] The justice that God is working for among us does not rest satisfied with simple welfare transfers. It requires whatever is necessary to enable everyone to *participate* in society as full members in ways appropriate to their dignity as God's loved children. It requires the development of a social context in which all who want them can find jobs that enable them to express themselves and develop their talents, to provide for their families basic needs, and to contribute to the common good.

The normal way to speak about issues of justice in our culture is in the language of "rights." And so the pastoral calls on us all to recognize as fundamental human rights those social contexts or conditions that are necessary for everyone to participate in society in ways that accord with their sacred human dignity. These economic rights include the rights to a job; to food, clothing, and shelter; to adequate healthcare; to education and leisure; and to security in old age. These are as fully human rights as our civil rights, and we need a national commitment to institutionalize and protect them.[20]

Implications for Healthcare

The implications of this analysis and theological interpretation are multiple and far reaching. As they begin to shape our outlook and decisions, the church's influence on the economy—and on healthcare economics as a result—will be extensive.

Already the pastoral has succeeded in turning the nation's attention once again to the poor and unemployed. At a time when the national mood favors ignoring them and shunting them aside, the church has legitimated and demanded serious debate over how to help the poor by transforming our socio-economic system. It is providing the context within which their specific healthcare needs can at least get a hearing. In addition, the programs for implementing the pastoral will help to generate a political constituency and produce political advocacy for economic rights—that broad base of economic conditions and opportunities necessary to enable all citizens to participate fully and productively in society. Those rights, of course, include the right to adequate health protection and care.[21]

Efforts to implement the pastoral will also be directed toward transforming the cultural bases that severely limit all current efforts to alleviate the economic crisis. There will be efforts to overcome our exaggerated individualism and rebuild community values through education and through experiments in participative management, workplace democracy, and local, regional, national, and international collaboration.[22] Vibrant and involved communities are the essential foundation for healthy healthcare economics.

It seems reasonable to infer, also, that if these efforts are somewhat successful and the nation begins to reach out to the poor and needy more during this "Exile" period of its history, there will be increasing pressure to contain healthcare costs. There will also be continuing pressure on healthcare institutions to gear their development and services to meet the specific needs of local communities better—and especially the needs of the poor in those communities. These pressures should combine to continue the reorientation of healthcare away from its heavy investment in "high-tech" acute care toward more comprehensive programs emphasizing health education and primary and preventive care.

Finally, the church will continue to press on the national consciousness the awareness that these issues are *global*, not national, in scope. At this time of "Exile" when we feel as a nation that we are losing our grip on economic security—indeed, on life as we have known it for several decades—it will be hard to be asked to let go further to embrace more of the poor and suffering of the world. Yet, paradoxically, that is the price of our liberation from Exile: renewal of the selfless compassion shown by the good Samaritan, a radically new national commitment to the sisterhood and brotherhood of all people.

The conversion we are being called to is not easy or attractive, at least not at first glance. We have lost touch with the richness of the deeper values we are being called back to. But reality will keep forcing itself on us. God can be inexorable. And as our understanding of what is happening grows, we can hope to see growing interest in creative ways to share our healthcare resources with the global poor.[23] It is obvious that this would affect healthcare economics in major ways.

Influence Through Integrity

My third point is that the church's influence on the economy in general and on healthcare economics in specific rests on the integrity with which it models the justice it calls for. This insight first appeared in the church's social teaching more than 15 years ago. The pastoral puts it this way:

> All the moral principles that govern the just operation of any economic endeavor apply to the church and its agencies and institutions; indeed the church should be exemplary. The Synod of Bishops in 1971 worded this challenge most aptly: "While the church is bound to give witness to justice, she recognizes that anyone who ventures to speak to people about justice must first be just in their eyes. Hence, we must undertake an examination of the modes of acting and of the possessions and lifestyle found within the church herself."[24]

The fifth chapter of the pastoral attempts to spell out some of the specific elements of the church's commitment to be a model of economic justice and to collaborate in creating a just economic order in which all will be treated with dignity.[25]

It is not necessary here to review the contents of that fifth chapter and conjecture about its potential impact.[26] Catholic healthcare providers are the most direct presence of the church, the people of God, in healthcare. They represent its most direct influence on healthcare economics. So it seems more valuable to devote the final reflections of this chapter to some of the pastoral's implications for healthcare institutions and systems.

Employers

The most obvious set of considerations centers on pay scales and benefits. In general, the church is notorious for the wages it pays. In the wake of this pastoral letter, all church institutions should be asking seriously how just its wage and benefit scales are. One healthcare system recently came to the embarrassing realization that some of its lower-paid and parttime employees did not receive health benefits. They were medically indigent and unable to get the care they needed to stay on the job. A new insight was gained into the demands of the preferential option for the poor. The CEO of another system began to see that the salary and incentive program it was introducing for top management served the reigning corporate value system and reflected no consciousness of the poor. Nor was there any comparable system for its wage workers. What are the demands of biblical justice with its preferential option for the poor at the *upper* end of the health system?

Lifestyle

These two experiences are important to reflect on. They raise the question of personal and corporate lifestyle, one of the important minor themes of the pastoral. A few years ago I lived in one of the most exclusive areas of a major city. The more I traveled, speaking about economic justice and concern for the poor, the more uncomfortable I became with the luxury of my living context. I am beginning to observe the same discomfort in healthcare documents now as they encourage, for example, the selection of meeting places and style more in accord with a preferential option for the poor.[27] That type of witness can be very impressive and effective. One high-priced consultant who was moved by the pastoral and by efforts he sees to live out its vision now cuts his fees dramatically when the meetings he attends are held in poor surroundings rather than luxury hotels. In effect, he is joining efforts to change the reigning corporate culture and values.

The pastoral asks that all members of the community and all its institutions reevaluate our lifestyle in the light of the needs of the global poor. From meeting locations to the quality of paper we print on to office furniture to salaries and benefits available to those on the bottom and those on the top, we must reflect prayerfully on all the everyday ways we express our identity and mission.

Being among the wealthiest 2 or 3 percent of the world's population, major healthcare administrators in the United States must reflect honestly and carefully on how they can take the most effective leadership in embodying a preferential option for the economically poor. An old slogan captures the call of the pastoral, the call that lurks in our own feelings of uneasiness as we try to discern the limits of our ability to serve the poor: we must find ways—personally and institutionally—to live more simply so that others may simply live. We must accept the possibility of being less well-heeled so that others may simply be healed.

Hiring

An institution's values are reflected in and shaped by its key personnel. Do the personnel and leadership in Catholic healthcare institutions reflect our belief in the equal and sacred dignity of people of all races and both genders? Do hiring processes enable them to find people who share this vision of justice and are committed to working for a more just society? If not, they run the very real risk of having the reigning economic vision and values of the nation's graduate and professional schools and corporate structures shape their institutional life and policies no matter what the rhetoric of their vision statements professes.

Management Structures

This justice vision requires participative management structures and practices in which everyone has some effective say in the decisions affecting the work environment. As I suggested in my first point, such structures can unleash the experience, creativity, and wisdom of thousands of workers and bring them to the service of the system's life and mission. In doing that, it will enable them to grow and develop and to discover in their work more meaning and sense of vocation.

Investments

Investments provide another matter for reflection. Do investment policies take as their primary guiding priority that—to use the pastoral's words—they *"should be specially directed to benefit those who are poor or economically insecure"*?[28] This priority, if modeled by church institutions, is sure to influence the economy and our culture. It clearly implies that return on investment is not the only ethical issue involved in financial decisions. There are other, usually more important, bottom lines to consider. As this realization grows in the churches, more resources are being developed to help institutions make more responsible investment decisions.[29]

Collaboration

The commitment to regional and national collaboration with other healthcare institutions and systems seems an excellent embodiment of the pastoral's call for "A New American Experiment in Partnership for the Public Good." It is especially welcome in contrast to the more competitive approaches of some Catholic healthcare institutions, which, in their search for financial security, have driven local clinics, hospices, and other long-standing community service projects out of business.

The spirit of the pastoral would certainly encourage extending collaborative efforts beyond the healthcare arena as well. Catholic healthcare's corporate strength makes it an important actor—along with businesses, churches, governments, and community organizations—in rebuilding our communities and our sense of commitment to the common good. Local and regional revitalization require extensive collaboration—and have important implications for healthcare and healthcare economics. What ways might Catholic systems and institutions take more effective leadership in stimulating this type of collaboration?

Community Relations

I have been wondering for sometime now whether the growing advertising budgets of healthcare institutions do not reflect a conventional sales approach to competing for market share. If so, I suspect that at least some of the money would be better spent on community organizers who could help local citizens rebuild a sense of community identity and identify their true community healthcare needs. I suspect that would generate much deeper community loyalty than passive "consumer satisfaction."

As these last reflections imply, the integrity of the witness of Catholic systems demands that they break out of the confines of their specializations in medicine and healthcare management. The problems they face in the healthcare economy are symptoms of the deeper economic transition and cultural disease our nation is caught up in. If they want to do more than treat the symptoms, they must support and advocate broader economic and cultural change. They must be concerned about job training and job programs targeted to the long term unemployed and the poor. They must continue and expand their commitments to healthcare as a basic human right by publicly supporting the full panoply of economic rights the pastoral calls for.

Finally, they must continue to think and plan with the planet as their backdrop. To be faithful to the Christian call to justice, we all must continue to expand our international vision

181

and outreach, making our identity as global citizens more central to our consciousness and activity. We are sisters and brothers to all people of the earth. We must guard, in our outreach, against cultural imperialism—that we do not go in as "experts" and create small images of ourselves around the world. But that is not an impossible task; it should not hold us back. The international outreach programs of many institutions and systems can open the hearts and minds of the personnel who participate in them, the institutions they come from and return to, the systems as a whole (eventually), and through all these a much broader community throughout the regions they serve. If these programs contribute to this, church influence (through the participating institutions) will be significant indeed.

Conclusion

These are just several of the economic pastoral's implications for our personal lives and institutional commitments. Many more are sure to arise in the ongoing struggle with these issues in the months and years ahead.

What is the church's influence in healthcare economics? It is the influence of a pastoral statement formulated out of the best community resources. It is the influence generated by revitalizing the church community and encouraging active involvement in the community's discernment of truth and pursuit of justice. It is the influence that comes from helping its members see the economic and cultural forces at work and recognize their religious significance. It is the influence that will flow from the integrity of our personal and institutional witness to the faith we embrace and the justice we pursue in every dimension of life.

We are in a period of extremely rapid change, but opportunities are massive. If, as I believe, this is an historical transition as significant as the Industrial Revolution, then we have the opportunity and the vocation to help shape a major new era, to try to find ways to make the world we are moving into more just than the one we are leaving. It is an exciting and a sacred challenge, one in which every person's talents and commitment are needed.

Footnotes
1. This chapter is a revision of an address by James E. Hug, SJ, given to the Third Annual Mercy Health Services Leadership Forum.
2. For more on this theme, see James E. Hug, SJ, and Rose Marie Scherschel, *Social Revelation*, Center of Concern, Washington, DC, 1988.
3. *Economic Justice for All: Pastoral Letter on Catholic Social Teaching and the U.S. Economy*, National Conference of Catholic Bishops, U.S. Catholic Conference, Washington, DC, 1986, #10.
4. *Economic Justice for All: Pastoral Letter on Catholic Social Teaching and the U.S. Economy*, #141. The pastoral cites studies by M. Harvey Brenner, P.H. Ellison, S.V. Kasl, and S. Cobb; L. E. Kopolow and F. M. Ochber; and D. Shaw. See footnote 9 to Chapter III of the letter.
5. *Economic Justice for All: Pastoral Letter on Catholic Social Teaching and the U.S. Economy*, #21. The quotation within the quotation is from the Second Vatican Council's *Pastoral Constitution on the Church in the Modern World #43*, in Walter M. Abott, SJ, The Documents of Vatican II, America Press, New York, 1966, p. 242.
6. I infer this from personal experience and from what appears to be a clearly analogous study by Jon Wisman in which he argues that hierarchical corporations that minimize participation by workers in decision making are actually acculturating them to subservience rather than self-reliance, critical thinking, and democratic involvement. See "Economic Reform for Humanity's Greatest Struggle," Council on International and Public Affairs, New York, 1986. Wisman cites a study by Lorraine B. Blank, who found that workers who own and control their own firms tend to become more active in both local politics and in voluntary organizations. See "The Impact of Workplace Participation: A Multivariate Analysis," PhD dissertation, The American University, Washington DC, 1985.
7. *Economic Justice for All: Pastoral Letter on Catholic Social Teaching and the U.S. Economy*, #11.
8. Lance Contrucci, "To Buy Is to Indulge a Yen," *New York Times* April 27, 1987, p. A19.
9. Ward Morehouse and David Dembo, *Joblessness and the Pauperization of Work in America*, Council on International and Public Affairs, New York, November 1986. This is one of a series of quarterly reports issued by the council (777 United Nations Plaza, New York, NY 10017). See also Lance Compa, "So We Have More Jobs—Low-Paid, Part-Time Ones," *The Washington Post*, 1987. The article reports on a Joint Economic Committee reported by Barry Bluestone of the University of Massachusetts and Bennett Harrison of MIT.
10. *Economic Justice for All: Pastoral Letter on Catholic Social Teaching and the U.S. Economy*, #21.
11. See, for example, the *Vision and Directional Statement* of Mercy Health Services, Farmington Hills, MI, 1986.
12. *Economic Justice for All: Pastoral Letter on Catholic Social Teaching and the U.S. Economy*, #22. See Peter Berger, Brigitte Berger, and Hansfried Kellner, *The Homeless Mind: Modernization and Consciousness*, Vintage, New York, 1974.
13. The automobile industry is only one recent example.
14. *Economic Justice for All: Pastoral Letter on Catholic Social Teaching and the U.S. Economy*, #30-40.

15. See Ralph W. Klein, *Israel in Exile: A Theological Interpretation,* Fortress Press, Philadelphia, 1979.
16. *Economic Justice for All: Pastoral Letter on Catholic Social Teaching and the U.S. Economy,* #41-52.
17. For a good discussion of these parables, see the article by Dennis Hamm, SJ, "Economic Policy and the Uses of Scripture," *America,* vol. 152, no. 17, May 4, 1985, pp. 368-371.
18. *Economic Justice for All: Pastoral Letter on Catholic Social Teaching and the U.S. Economy,* #44.
19. *Economic Justice for All: Pastoral Letter on Catholic Social Teaching and the U.S. Economy,* #56-78.
20. *Economic Justice for All: Pastoral Letter on Catholic Social Teaching and the U.S. Economy,* #77-95.
21. *Economic Justice for All: Pastoral Letter on Catholic Social Teaching and the U.S. Economy,* #80.
22. *Economic Justice for All: Pastoral Letter on Catholic Social Teaching and the U.S. Economy,* Chapter 4.
23. For more on this, see Chapter 10, "Generating a Truly *Catholic* Response in Difficult Times."
24. *Economic Justice for All: Pastoral Letter on Catholic Social Teaching and the U.S. Economy,* #347. This quotation from the 1971 Synod of Bishops is taken from the document Justice in the World, #40.
25. *Economic Justice for All: Pastoral Letter on Catholic Social Teaching and the U.S. Economy,* #326-365.
26. For a concise summary of its contents (and of the whole pastoral), see James E. Hug, SJ, *For All the People,* U.S. Catholic Conference, Washington, DC, 1986.
27. For example, "Corporate policy at the association, system, and local facility level should ensure that travel, meetings, buildings, and entertainment reflect the Catholic healthcare mission and be appropriately modest. *"No Room in the Marketplace: The Health Care of the Poor,* The Catholic Health Association of the United States, St. Louis, 1986, p. 19. In August 1985 the task force on the care of the poor of the Bon Secours Health System had recommended: "Corporate policy should assure that travel, meetings, buildings, and entertainment reflect the mission of Catholic healthcare, i.e., be appropriately modest. There should be a system-wide understanding of the importance of the corporate witness to simplicity and ongoing evaluation of style and image in relation to the corporate policy. *"Bon Secours Means Good Help to Those in Need,* Columbia, MD: Bon Secours Health System, Inc., 1985, p. 7.
28. *Economic Justice for All: Pastoral Letter on Catholic Social Teaching and the U.S. Economy,* #92 (emphasis in the text).
29. One of the most well known is ICCR, the Interfaith Center on Corporate Responsibility, 475 Riverside Drive, Room 566, New York, NY 10115. ICCR works with another organization at the same address, the Clearinghouse on Alternate Investments. IRRC, the Investor Responsibility Research Center, Inc., works out of Suite 600, 1755 Massachusetts Ave., NW, Washington, DC, 20036. In the midwest is NCCRI, the National Catholic Coalition for Responsible Investment, 1016 N. Ninth Street, Milwaukee, WI 53233. It is affiliated with ICCR. A number of newsletters provide information and resource lists for possible alternative investments. One is *CATALYST: Investing in Social Change*

(available from P.O. Box 364, Worcester, VT 05682). Two recent books are helpful: Steven D. Lydenberg, Alice Tepper Marlin, Sean O'Brien Strub, and the Council on Economic Priorities *Rating America's Corporate Conscience: A Provocative Guide to the Companies Behind the Products You Buy Every Day,* Addison-Wesley, Reading, MA, 1987, and Amy L. Domini and Peter D. Kinder, *Ethical Investing: How To Make Profitable Investments without Sacrificing Your Principles,* Reading, MA; Addison-Wesley, 1984.

Reflection Questions

1. This chapter explores the question of the church's influence in healthcare economics by looking at the U.S. pastoral letter on the economy: its process, its analyses, and the integrity of our response to it.

   - Do you know of any programs planned to promulgate the pastoral throughout the church? What are they? How might you find more information?

   - What do you understand by the image of the church as the People of God?

   - How can participative processes be made more operational in healthcare institutions and systems?

   - Can you suggest ways we might be able to experiment with participative management, workplace democracy, and local, regional, national, and international collaboration? Can you cite examples where such are already operational?

   - What connections do you see between religious and moral values and economic and cultural forces?

   - What can individuals or groups do to influence the adjustment of the world economy so that the poor's rights are protected?

   - Can you cite examples of the sense of the whole being lost due to specialization and the division of labor? What are they?

   - What can be done to counter the social passivity of our times?

   - Can you list the personal economic rights enumerated in this chapter?

   - Is it realistic to think that we might be able to influence a national commitment to institutionalize and protect all people's human rights? How might we approach it?

   - In the development and planning of your institution, are your local community's specific needs taken into account? How? Whose voices are listened to?

   - Can you cite examples other than those noted in the chapter that would be visible extensions and applications of the values the pastoral expresses?

   - Do you experience any discrepancies when you examine your personal lifestyle and your institution(s) hiring, management structure, and investments compared with the values expressed in the pastoral?

· 12 ·

Ministry to a People on the Edge of Exile: Reflections on the Contemporary Call of U.S. Catholic Chaplains[1]

James E. Hug, SJ

As we reflect on ministry, it is important to reflect on the fact that we are participating in one of the most significant periods of recorded history. We have stepped into a global socioeconomic transition that rivals the Industrial Revolution for its importance and far-reaching implications. The current tensions within healthcare—as in practically any of the social institutions served by chaplains—can trace their roots to the forces generating this transition.

Such significant change, as unsettling as it invariably is, brings with it a major call to conversion. Breakthroughs in nuclear physics, the development of microchips, and now the probability of high-temperature superconductors have contributed to the emergence of a Kairos—a sacred time in which God makes available the possibility of radically graced transformation, both personal and social. The challenge facing us is how to participate in shaping the emerging world so that it will be more just, more revealing of the Reign of God among us.

This historical context makes it an exciting and important time to look seriously at chaplaincy and pastoral care—to celebrate their achievements and to reflect on their roles and challenges as participants in the contemporary *Kairos*.

Celebrating the Grace That Is

Twenty-five years ago, Pope John XXIII opened the first session of the Second Vatican Council. We all know what a land-mark that event was, what a sea change it signaled for the Catholic Church. By the time its final session opened in Fall 1965, the National Association of Catholic Chaplains had begun to meet in annual convention. The church and all its ministries were launched on a major renewal that has brought about remarkable changes in pastoral care. It has evolved from a relatively simple and straight-forward sacramental ministry in priests' hands into a complex and rich variety of spiritual ministries requiring mixed ecumenical teams. It has grounded itself in experience rather than church law and teaching.

It has not been an easy transition, however. Through these years, pastoral ministers have taken on the often painful task of learning to deal with human feelings and not just dismiss them as biased or signs of weakness or as temptations. They first had to learn to get to know and appreciate their own feelings; next they learned those of their clients, their clients' families, their institu-tion's staffs, and their colleagues in ministry. They have had to learn—and then to help others learn—to discern God's revelation in those feelings. They have had to learn anew to face disease, grief, aging, and death—this time on a consciously experiential level—and to discover God's personal word in them. And they have had to learn to help others do the same.

They have had to struggle with stress and burnout. They have returned again and again to such difficult questions as the type of theological formation they need and how pastoral theology and ministry should relate to moral theology with its judgments of right and wrong in such difficult areas as organ transplants, surrogate motherhood, withdrawing life support systems, and acquired immune deficiency syndrome (AIDS). In recent years some have explored the role of prayer and faith in healing. Others have begun to work with dreams. Important arenas of ministry have opened to women, and pioneering work in the mutuality of women and men in ministry is being undertaken.

Through these years they have had to rethink their professional image and even their very identity.[2] These are traumatic experiences. There are, I am sure, many wounded and anxious people searching to find meaning and direction in their pastoral ministry today.

These significant changes in the whole range of pastoral ministries have resulted from a variety of influences. They have not been the simple result of an obedient implementation of a Vatican II directive that pastoral care should develop in these ways. Through the open windows of the Council, the major intellectual and social currents of the 19th and 20th centuries—psychology, sociology, and the rise of historical consciousness — blew into the church. Psychology proved especially fruitful and appealing for those engaged in pastoral ministries, and many of the advances made in this field are due to the creative application of psychological insight in ministry.

Similar developments occurred everywhere in the church's life. Contemporary thought fertilized the burgeoning renewals underway in scripture studies, liturgy, and theology, bringing new energy and insight. We rediscovered the God of Love so central to the scriptures—the God who is present to and involved with our experience and history.

As we all pursued the insights and followed the guidance of the Holy Spirit as faithfully as we could, we gradually found our energies refocused and our ministries redirected to the heart of Christian life: helping each other receive God's love, discern God's presence and invitation in our experience, and respond in faith and love. This became the key to pastoral ministry: helping people discern God's call in their experience.

The Kairos of Today:
The Social Revelation of Exile

There is, indeed, a great deal to celebrate in this brief history. Yet even as the struggle goes on to develop the insights and the complex sense of ministry that have begun to emerge through the contributions of psychology and theology, other external forces—beyond those of psychology, sociology, and historical consciousness—demand our attention. It is an uneasy time for healthcare and all social service ministries.

Life-threatening economic pressures have brought on a crisis in healthcare. In an effort to contain healthcare costs, the federal government has instituted diagnosis-related groups (DRGs) and cut back eligibility for a variety of social programs. Third party payers have embraced DRGs and have begun hard bargaining designed to cut their healthcare expenses. Healthcare is increasingly being pushed into the marketplace.

Healthcare institutions have responded by tightening up business practices, consolidating, and trying to develop attractive new "marketable" services. The new emphasis on the business side of healthcare has given rise to the "healthcare industry" mentality. The sick are no longer "patients" or "clients," but "healthcare consumers." Healthcare services are now "product lines." Concern for service of community needs is yielding center stage to considerations of profitability, competitiveness, and economic efficiency. The language of the business corporation is pervading the healthcare atmosphere.[3]

The danger in the rise of this kind of metaphor is that it threatens to subordinate everything else. Pastoral care is no longer an obvious value; it must prove its marketability, its potential as a financial asset. I do not mean to question the fact that some forms of pastoral care are "eminently marketable." I merely want to point out that as soon as we enter this conversation, we have entered an arena in which business values are considered the criteria of evaluation—"the bottom line."

These economic pressures are forcing us to ask some very fundamental questions, questions that press to the very identity of healthcare. What part does chaplaincy play in healthcare? What part does Catholic healthcare play in the larger healthcare picture? The rise of the for-profit healthcare systems have been a major challenge. How, honestly, does Catholic healthcare differ? The recent CHA study on Catholic identity in healthcare is a first effort to respond, but adequate answers remain far away.[4]

The questions do not stop there, however. What part does healthcare play in the nation's economy? What part should it play? What part does the economy play in U.S. social and political life and culture? And what part do all these factors play in the life and health of people chaplains minister to?

If the developments in ministry in the last 25 years have opened us to God in personal and interpersonal experience, these questions seem to indicate the agenda for the next 25 years. We must develop the skills and ability to discern God's presence, activity, and invitation in life's social, economic, political, and cultural dimensions. We are called to learn to read the *social revelation* present in our lives, the Word of God in the *signs of the times.*[5]

In the last two decades, the concern with social revelation and justice issues has been left to the social activists, those with interests and skills in social ministry. Now practically the full array of social justice issues are arising in the heart of even the most intimate pastoral care situations. We are being forced to recognize that everyone is *simultaneously* engaged at personal, interpersonal, and societal levels. These levels cannot be artificially separated to satisfy our areas of ministerial specialization. To be effective ministers of Jesus, we must be alert and responsive to the revelation of God in all the dimensions of life in which we, and those to whom we minister, participate.

During Holy Week of 1986, I visited a peasant family displaced from their land by the military in El Salvador. They were living in a camp on the edge of San Salvador without home or land of their own. The father of the family said to those of us who were visiting, "They bomb our land. They burn our crops. They drive us from our land and our villages. They round us up and take us where we don't want to go. Then they give us a little food and lecture us on how they are our friends!"

In that context the Archdiocese of San Salvador has decided to refuse all food and medicine offered by the military and U.S. A.I.D. for the displaced poor and sick. It is clear that to accept them and channel them to the poor would make the church a cooperator in the government's pacification plan. It would be hidden from no one. This family and their friends would know immediately. They would conclude that once again the church hierarchy was aligning itself with the rich and powerful. "They bomb our land and take us where we do not want to go. They give us a little food. The church calls it Christian charity offered in the name of our God, and we hear lectures on how they are our friends."

In the history of Christian ministry, feeding the hungry and caring for the sick have been considered corporal works of mercy—good things taken in themselves. What the father of that family and, increasingly, our own context are teaching us is that no simple activity like that is ever "taken in itself." It is part of a larger complex social reality and has its real significance within that reality.

Now even chaplains must ask themselves whether their ministry might be just a small humanizing touch being used to legitimate or market an increasingly dehumanizing technological business that reflects and responds to our national fear of death and our disregard for the poor.

Our deep cultural fascination with youth is the reverse side of a profound anxiety over death. One of the speakers at the 1987 Catholic Health Assembly said: "This generation will fight aging tooth and nail. The [baby] boomers like their youth so much they'll do everything they can to take it with them to old age."[6]

Their concern for aging parents and their own aging promise to make their health concerns the most significant factor shaping healthcare over the next decade. They have the financial means to command the attention of healthcare institutions in our current market-driven atmosphere.[7] That promises to continue and to increase the commitment of disproportionately large percentages of our healthcare resources to the last few months and years of life.

What role will chaplains play in this scenario? Will they find themselves increasingly becoming counselors to the aging wealthy? Will they be a symbolic religious presence adding religious legitimacy to a healthcare system increasingly oriented to using the latest technology to salvage a few extra days or months for those who can afford to pay for them while millions of people nationally and billions globally go without attention to their most basic health needs?

This type of question challenges us to rethink chaplaincy, chaplaincy training, and certification. We need chaplains who are as aware of the role they play in their institutional setting as they are of their own feelings. We need chaplains with the skills to discern the *social* contexts of human suffering, disease, and death as well as the personal contexts. We need chaplains capable of reading God's *social* revelation and recognizing its presence in the intimate moments of personal suffering they are privileged to minister to.

I raise these not as so many new tasks for overworked chaplains to add to their agendas. I am not suggesting that now they must do "social justice things" too. I am not trying to hasten burnout! I am pointing to what I believe is our call as ministers in this *Kairos*. It is a call to a deeper awareness, a fuller consciousness of the reality we are *already* living. Each of us is now deeply immersed in a complex world of the personal, interpersonal, and societal dimensions. So is everyone with whom we interact. Every bit of ministry we do is already a form of social ministry. Not even the corporal and spiritual works of mercy can be simply "taken in themselves," isolated from their social context and role. What we are being called to now is a greater awareness of the role our actions truly play in the larger social picture. We are being called to more effective forms of pastoral ministry in our contemporary social context.

What, then, might it mean to minister with an awareness of the social, cultural, political, and economic contexts within which the ministerial encounter is taking place? What is the social experience, the social revelation of the people we deal with in pastoral care today in this country?

A People on the Edge of Exile

There is an emerging intuition in the U.S. church, reflected in the recent pastoral letters of the U.S. bishops on peace and the economy, that we are a people on the edge of exile. Both letters suggest that some of the most helpful biblical texts for throwing light on our contemporary experience and helping us interpret it in faith come from Israel's experience of exile in Babylon.[8]

At first it is not so clear why we might be considered a people undergoing an exile experience. The U.S. remains the most powerful nation in the world. There are some signs of economic recovery. We are not experiencing literal conquests or deportations. Yet if we probe the notion of exile a bit further, the idea becomes more plausible.

Old Testament scholar Ralph Klein has written:
the questions posed by the exilic age or perceived by the biblical writers were so acute and so modern—questions of identity and the grounds for hope, ques-

tions about who or what is the cause of Israel's malaise, questions about the continuing validity of symbols and symbol systems, questions for and in a time of radical change, questions for those who are rootless or whose future seems fruitless and fraught with con-flict.[9]

Are those contemporary questions in the United States? It seems to me they are. As I look back over the last 25 years in which pastoral ministry has been developing so fruitfully, I see a series of trau-matic events that have struck at our sense of national identity, leaving us a wounded people.

Traumatic History

The period begins with a popular, energetic, idealistic, young president leading a nation that saw itself as the carrier of Judeo-Christian and democratic values for the world. It was a proud time. He was brutally and senselessly assassinated. In the years follow John Kennedy's death, we gradually came to discover our involvement in Vietnam and in Chile as violations of our proudest principles. The civil rights movement challenged us to face injustice in our own society. Prophetic leaders like Martin Luther King and Robert Kennedy were killed. The women's movement showed us that as a society we did not even know how to enter the most fundamental human relationship without perpetuating oppression. Watergate gave us corruption at the highest levels of our public institutions. It left us with the pitiful image of our presi-dent pleading that he was not a crook and resigning in disgrace. Oil crises in the early and late 1970s taught us our addiction to cheap energy and our dependence on those who produce it. The heritage of the crisis was nearly a decade of simultaneous economic stagnation and inflation and an international debt crisis that threatens the global financial system to this day. Nixon's successor, Gerald Ford, was a conciliator who brought some healing to the nation; but he soon won the image of incompetence. The most powerful nation of the world had a leader who couldn't walk and chew gum at the same time.

Jimmy Carter experimented with a new role for the United States in the world. He saw us as a partner among equals on the world stage. He modeled a new relationship between the sexes in his marriage. He attempted to ground foreign policy in concern for human rights. But Iran took U.S. hostages, and the nation felt impotent. Carter was attacked by Ronald Reagan for weakness and rejected by voters who wanted to believe Reagan's message that we could return to the sense of ourselves that we had when this era began. What we got instead was a massive military build-up, erosion of environmental safeguards, cuts in social programs, the highest unemployment, and the most bank and farm failures since the Great Depression, the rapid emergence of the United States as the greatest debtor nation in the history of the world, and the worst stock market crash in history. Moreover, we have been awash in the corruption and deceit of the Iran/Contra affair.

Who are we as a nation? We thought we knew in 1960, and we were proud of who we thought we were. But in the last 25 years, each element of that identity has come under serious attack. Vietnam and Chile shattered our sense of our place and role in the world. Watergate, financial scandals on Wall Street, and the Iran/Contra affair have undermined our sense of moral upright-ness and brought into question the practicality and sincerity of our stated ideals. Our economic slide has challenged our sense of ourselves as creative and competent people. The civil rights move-ment and the women's movement have shown up our ability to form lifegiving relationships. The slipping economy and the global nuclear threat question our ability to provide a better world for the next generation.

National Identity Crisis

If we stop and reflect on what has been happening, it becomes clear that the social supports and institutional under-pinnings for all the dimensions of identity that Erik Erikson has taught us have been battered during this period.[10] It is a time of serious national identity crisis. We are a people in need of help to reflect on our experience, to understand it in the light of our faith, and to put ourselves back together again in ways that might be more faithful to our deepest ideals. We need a prophet, a pastoral minister. Or, perhaps better, we need wounded healers who have experienced a loss of their sense of identity and are engaging in the struggle to deepen a more constructive and lifegiving identity for the changed situation in which we live. We need the help of a truly redemptive vision to guide us at this delicate time in the history of our national psyche.

Ronald Reagan has tried to provide that vision and has been an unfortunately effective prophet. He has held up the vision of the 1950s:

- Our place in the world? "The United States is indeed Number One, and the free world wants us to act like it. We are ready to fight for freedom [and so we stage Grenada] and we support those who do [the "Freedom Fighters" in Nicaragua and Afghanistan]."
- Our moral uprightness? "Don't confuse us with the Soviet Union! They are the Evil Empire."
- Creativity and competence? "Let's get back to basics, work harder, increase productivity, compete harder. We can and must trust our technology. It will bring us economic dominance once again, and secure peace."
- The loss of ideals? "We need to reclaim the ideals that made the nation great—the free market, democracy, the myth of the self-reliant individual." Reagan's presidential portrait is in stark contrast to those of the other presidents in the National Portrait Gallery. It depicts him as a cowboy on his ranch.
- Oppressive relations between races? "Now our civil rights legislation creates discrimination against whites and generates dependency in blacks. These laws should be eliminated."
- Oppressive relations between the sexes? "A tempest in a teapot! Ron and Nancy happily model a traditional marriage relationship."
- "America is back. There will be a better tomorrow." The message is offered with a grandfatherly smile by a person seemingly at peace with himself.

The whole picture is an Eriksonian dream. It speaks to all levels of identity formation and stabilization. But it holds the promise of becoming a national nightmare. It is not a vision that illuminates our reality; it is one that masks its deeper forces and orientation. It worships an individualism that refuses to face the loss of a common moral vision and concern for the common good that are eroding our communities.[11] It makes us comfortable with our prejudices. It glosses over the fact that the technological development it supports in production, communications, and transportation will continue to replace jobs and make it easier for corporations to move their production facilities, abandoning our cities and towns in search of cheaper labor elsewhere in the world. It ignores the severe ecological damage resulting from dangerous industrial practices and high intensity, high tech farming techniques. The loss of family farms has reached crisis proportions, and with it comes the death of small town America.

A brighter future? Economic recovery? The same data showing declining unemployment reveal that practically all new jobs are at the low-paying end of the service sector. They are jobs at or near the poverty line that carry few, if any, benefits. This economic recovery is not eliminating poverty or healthcare indigence. Rather, it seems to cement them in place as our future. The gap between the wealthy and the poor is growing; the middle class is shrinking. The exile continues: jobs are being exiled to the Third World; the land is being exiled to absentee corporate control; the wealth is being exiled into the hands of fewer and fewer people. The young and talented are being exiled to serve the centers of wealth and power. Those who have felt the suffering respond to the theme of exile.

Challenge to Ministry in a Time of Exile

What does all this have to do with the daily ministry of chaplains and other pastoral ministers? I believe it is present in some form in every person they encounter—if only you have the eyes to see.

It is present in the *patients* and residents of their institutions whose illnesses and destructive behavior have been caused or aggravated by the conditions of our social context. Data show that a local plant closing can generate notable increases in heart disease, hypertension, ulcers, respiratory diseases and allergic reactions, alcoholism, spouse abuse, child abuse, and infant mortality. Poverty breeds malnutrition and a host of infant diseases. We have even seen a recurrence of Third World diseases such as marasmus and kwashiorkor in the United States in recent years. Pollution and radiation are filling cancer wards.[12]

Some patients are seeking healthcare only when they are quite sick. When people are too poor to pay for healthcare—or too poor to take time off from work or family responsibilities to get it—they put it off as long as possible, hoping that they will get better without it. They are staying less time and leaving the hospital sicker because of the economic pressures on healthcare institutions.

The unemployed and underemployed suffer from feelings of inadequacy, failure, and depression. As the economic pastoral points out,

> It is a deep conviction of American culture that work is central to the freedom and well-being of people. The unemployed often come to feel they are worthless and without a productive role in society. Each day they are unemployed our society tells them: We don't need your talent. We don't need your initiative. We don't need you. Unemployment takes a terrible toll on the health and stability of both individuals and families.[13]

Or, if pastoral ministers are not encountering these realities, that too requires social discernment. Why not? Are they seeing fewer and fewer poor? Are the poor being excluded from care by marketplace pressures? The challenge to pastoral ministry today is to discover how to discern the social revelation present in each of these contexts and how to minister more effectively as a result.

This social context is also present in an institution's staff. Staff members are frequently under pressure now because of reduced personnel and increased workloads. They labor, too, under pressure of increased job insecurity. Millions of people in this nation hover on the brink of poverty; it is only one serious disease, one job loss, one divorce, or one death in the family away. Those pressures contribute to a host of stress-related diseases. The impact of the global economy, mediated by the marketplace pressures on healthcare, is being felt at nursing stations and on kitchen and maintenance crews across the nation. What is the revelation here? What are we being called to in pastoral ministry?

The global social context is also present in the *institutional policies* governing our institutions. Are they increasingly being dominated by business values and priorities? Are there moves to reduce pay scales and fight unions? Are there subtle moves to reduce the numbers of medically indigent treated? Are there growing pressures to justify every service by market values? Can

198

employees participate in decisions that affect their workplace and the care they give? Are wages just? Are administrators starting to talk about "biting the bullet" and limiting healthcare to the poor without questioning their own six-figure incomes, expensive resort-based seminars, and so on?

These observations and questions just scratch the surface. We have learned through the years to approach each person with psychological sensitivities and questions so that we can minister more effectively to their true religious needs. We are just beginning to develop similar social sensitivities and learn the right social questions with which to probe.

We have learned, too, the healing power of healthy human relationships and the importance of modeling them in our ministry. We still must learn how to model healthy and healing relationships on the institutional, systemic, and societal levels. If we cannot model them, our healing social word will be empty and our ministry to others crippled. One of the crucial tasks awaiting the leadership of pastoral care teams as we face the challenge of discerning social revelation is the task of helping our institutions and systems reflect on our corporate experience, interpret it, and respond to it in the light of our faith.

Chaplains of the Exile

If the motif of exile is helpful for understanding the type of fundamental human experience we are going through as a people, the forms of pastoral ministry that emerged in response to Israel's exile experience might help us to understand the challenge to pastoral ministry presented by this *Kairos*.

As is only natural, an immense amount of pastoral ministry went on in response to the trauma of Israel's exile. What did it mean that this could happen to God's Chosen People? Practically all the signs of God's special love for them were lost. The Promised Land was no longer theirs. Jerusalem lay in ruins. The Davidic monarchy was at an end. The Temple had been desecrated and destroyed. Was their God not as mighty as the God of the Babylonians? Had their God rejected them? Jeremiah, the author of the *Book of Lamentations*, the Deuteronomic Historian, the Priestly authors, Ezekiel, and Second Isaiah all came forward in ministry to help the people interpret the revelation of God in their societal experience.

199

As I reflect on these "Chaplains of the Exile," it occurs to me that they were working in different ways to facilitate the stages of death and dying for their people.[14]

Jeremiah

Jeremiah's primary ministry was to help Israel break through its *denial*. Even as the Israelite politicians were plotting revolution to escape Babylon's control, Jeremiah was walking through the streets of Jerusalem with a yoke on his shoulders. His symbolic word: "Face and accept the inevitable domination and exile." He had to fight the false prophets who were glibly promising peace and freedom. And once the exile came, he wrote to those taken off to Babylon telling them to settle in for a long stay. This exile was part of God's plan. His message was not without hope, however. In a final symbolic gesture, he bought land in Israel as a promise of future restoration.

In some cases, a socially conscious pastoral ministry will be called to similar responses. Are patients really facing what is happening in their social context and seeing its influence on their health? Or are they dealing with their stress by telling themselves they just have to work harder, compete more effectively, or get lucky?

Are staff and administrators facing what is happening in healthcare because of developments in the larger economy? Are they accepting the fact that their impending enslavement to those with market power cannot be averted by a little managerial tinkering and tightening up? Are they recognizing that their economic decisions and policies are religious issues that must be guided by faith? Are any of us facing honestly the call to conversion present in our context, a call to simpler lifestyles and expectations and to more communitarian values? Jeremiah's ministry to denial is badly needed today.

Lamentations

The author of *Lamentations* responded to the human need to *grieve*. The profound losses of home, land, and religious identity imposed by the exile required mourning. The *anger* that they stirred had to be addressed.

The same is true of the great losses being experienced in the United States. When an industrial plant closes in a blue collar neighborhood, more is lost than jobs. The community begins to grieve the loss of an entire way of life characterized by stable family and neighborhood, traditional values and forms of parenting, and middle class lifestyle.[15] When farmers lose their farms, they are forced out of the only way of life they have known, the freedom and closeness to nature that they love. And the small communities that they have built and that rely on their participation, their business, and their taxes are shaken. All too frequently, they collapse. When social services and healthcare are cut back, health, dignity, lifestyle, and hope all suffer.

Many among us need help in grieving our reality. We need to vent our rage and ask why this is happening to generous, dedicated, hard-working, and self-sacrificing people. Why is God letting this happen? Unless we face our grief and anger, we will continue to take it out on each other and the rest of the world.

The Deuteronomic Historian

The Deuteronomic Historian helped Israel move beyond its temptation to *bargain* so that it could look seriously at itself and its history. The books of *Deuteronomy, Joshua, Judges, 1* and *2 Samuel,* and *1* and *2 Kings* constitute a massive examination of conscience and confession of sin. They represent an effort to discover where Israel went wrong as a people, where they were unfaithful to their covenant with God, bringing their suffering on themselves.

Only when we have broken through our denial and vented our grief will we be able as a nation to enter on that kind of examination of conscience. The U.S. bishops have tried to begin that process with their pastoral letter on the economy. They have identified our cultural individualism and our loss of a common moral vision or sense of the common good.[16] These are rooted in an ideology of individual freedom that must be corrected and balanced by a renewal of community values.[17]

The bishops have highlighted the racism and sexism that still scar our national life.[18] They have pointed firmly to our exclusion of the poor from services and especially from full participation in society in ways that are in accord with their human dignity as children of God.[19] And they have challenged us to reevaluate our lifestyles—both personal and corporate—in the light of the basic needs of the poor locally and globally.[20]

It seems to me that we also must look seriously at how we have made idols of technology and the myth of "progress." We must question our fear of death that presses us to marshal all the most impressive forces of high technology to keep it at bay while ignoring the literally billions of inhabitants of this earth who do not have access to the most rudimentary medicines—and even lack clean water.

The Priestly Writers

The Priestly Writers had to contend with the exiles' depression and the Babylonians' belief that human beings were fundamentally evil. They were working with a people humiliated by defeat and living in slavery to a nation whose faith declared that humanity was the offspring of evil, defeated gods. The purpose of humanity was to do the work the gods did not want to do.

In that context the Priestly Writers developed the theology of the creation narratives of *Genesis* affirming the human person's profound dignity as the image of the one God. They recalled God's special concern for the poor expressed so clearly in the covenant made with Israel at Sinai. And they reminded the Israelites of God's fidelity to the covenant promises made to Noah and to Abraham and Sarah. They encouraged them to remain faithful to their identity, to maintain their worship, and not to succumb to the dominant culture around them.

These are some of the theological themes chosen by the U.S. bishops as most appropriate for us to reflect on today.[21] Every person has the profound dignity of a beloved child of God—not just those who are succeeding in the marketplace. The gifts of creation are meant to be shared to meet the needs of all, no matter what their race, gender, nationality, or achievement. These are words of healing for those in depression; they are words of prophetic challenge for those who are blind or insensitive to the needs of the poor and to the suffering caused by the shifting global forces in our contemporary *Kairos*.

On the institutional level, pastoral ministry in this Priestly tradition must challenge the cultural assumption that those who fail in our society fail because they are worthless, lazy, or evil.

A virulent form of social Darwinism has reasserted itself in recent years. We must call each other and our institutions—with their policies and corporate cultures—to fidelity to our true religious identity. We are—with all the people of creation—children of a loving God. We are called to see our work, whether in business or the social services or healthcare, as ministry. We must help each other and our institutions and systems remain faithful to that fundamental identity.

Ezekiel

Ezekiel, too, ministered to the *depressed* exiles in Babylon. Through the exotic description of his vision of God, he reminded them that God was present with them in Babylon. They had not been abandoned. They were being taken through an experience of death and resurrection by a God who could breathe new life into dry bones and write a new covenant on their hearts.

Second Isaiah

Second Isaiah's message echoes and expands on Ezekiel's. God is willing and able to forgive and build anew. Israel can *accept* this exile in hope. If they bear its suffering patiently— as the Suffering Servant—they will be a light to the nations and will one day return home in a new Exodus. The exile will have done its work, liberating them from the slavery of sinfulness that had bound them for too long.

There is no question that the American people need such a message of hope. Ronald Reagan's popularity bears eloquent testimony to it. All who would provide pastoral care to the people of our age must convey a word of true hope. It must not reflect an easy optimism, however. It must be a challenging hope based on purification through our experience of exile. It must be a hope written in the hearts of those who are willing to stand faithfully with the poor, rebuild our communities, and model just and healing relationships personally, institutionally, and systemically.

That witness could be very costly. The age of the Suffering Servant is not over either for individuals or for institutions or systems. But the promise is clear. Suffering borne in faith and love will be redemptive, a light to the nations. It will bear fruit in a "return" to the promised land of greater justice and peace.

Conclusion

There is a great deal to celebrate in the recent history of pastoral ministry and a great deal of challenge in its future. In some ways it is not a new challenge but an extension of the fundamental mission: *to help each other receive God's love, discern God's presence and invitation in our experience, and respond in faith and love.* It is a call to learn to discern and embrace all dimensions of God's revelation in the rich complexity of the *Signs of Our Times.* This is a critical period for our nation. We are a wounded people. Our identity crisis is painful and disorienting. It also contains the seeds of hope for radical conversion and societal healing, however. We need effective chaplains to this experience of exile, wounded healers who can walk with us and help us grow into a more Christ-like identity for today. We need effective pastoral care to help guarantee that this historic time of transition ushers in a more healthy, holy, and just global tomorrow.

Footnotes

1. This chapter is a revision of the Terrence Cardinal Cooke Memorial Lecture given by James E. Hug, SJ, at the annual convention of the National Association of Catholic Chaplains, Sept. 6, 1987.
2. Many of these developments have paralled developments in Christian spirituality and spiritual direction in the years since the Council. They, too have focused on the presence of God in personal experience and on the power of feelings and interpersonal relationships to carry contemporary revelation. Spiritual directors have come to describe themselves with a number of metaphors such as midwife or companion on the journey. The model for their ministry—as, in many ways, for yours—is the nondirective counselor. It is no longer the teacher or judge—images that governed the sense of identity of the spiritual director and the pastoral minister before the Council.
3. For more on this, see Chapter 2, "Catholic Healthcare: Competing and Complementary Models."
4. *The Dynamics of Catholic Identity in Healthcare: A Working Document,* The Catholic Health Association, St. Louis, 1987.
5. For more on this topic, see James E. Hug, SJ, and Rose Marie Scherschel, *Social Revelation: A Profound Challenge for Christian Spirituality,* Center of Concern, Washington, DC, 1987. This is one volume in a series of books on socially conscious spirituality entitled *Energies for Social Transformation.*
6. Kenneth Dychtwald, PhD, "Baby Boomers Changing Healthcare for Aging," *Health Progress,* July-August 1987, p. 70.
7. "The Elderly Will Shape Healthcare in the '90s," *Catholic Health World,* Aug. 15, 1987, p. 1, 4. The article describes the results of a Delphi study of more than 1,600 healthcare professionals conducted by Arthur Andersen & Co. and the American College of Healthcare Executives.

8. *Economic Justice for All: Pastoral Letter on Catholic Social Teaching and the U.S. Economy,* National Conference of Catholic Bishops, U.S. Catholic Conference, Washington, DC, 1986, #31. The section begins "After the exile . . . ." The theological reflection done on the exile experience is what is perceived as helpful for interpreting the revelation in our contemporary experience. *The Challenge of Peace: God's Promise and Our Response,* National Conference of Catholic Bishops, U.S. Catholic Conference, Washington, DC, 1983, #31. The exile is presented as the key turning point in their understanding of God and God's role in war and peace.

9. Ralph W. Klein, *Israel in Exile: A Theological Interpretation,* Fortress Press, Philadelphia, 1979, p. 7.

10. For the discussion of the social foundations of identity, see Erik Erikson, *Toys and Reasons: Stages in the Ritualization of Experience,* W. W. Norton & Co., New York, 1977, pp. 67-120.

11. See Robert N. Bellah, et al., *Habits of the Heart: Individualism and Commitment in American Life,* University of California Press, Berkeley, 1985. See also the U.S. bishops pastoral letter on the economy, ##22-27.

12. *Economic Justice for All: Pastoral Letter on Catholic Social Teaching and the U.S. Economy,* #141-143 with their footnote references. Also, see Isabel Wilkerson, "Infant Mortality: Frightful Odds in Inner City," *The New York Times,* June 26, 1987, pp. A1, A20.

13. *Economic Justice for All: Pastoral Letter on Catholic Social Teaching and the U.S. Economy,* #141.

14. Elisabeth Kubler-Ross, *On Death and Dying,* Macmillan New York, 1969.

15. I am relying here on the work of ethician John Raines with a blue-collar community in Philadelphia. For more, see John Raines, Lenora E. Berson, and David McI. Gracie, ed., *Community and Capital in Conflict: Plant Closings and Job Loss,* Temple University Press, Philadelphia, 1982.

16. *Economic Justice for All: Pastoral Letter on Catholic Social Teaching and the U.S. Economy,* ##21-27.

17. *Economic Justice for All: Pastoral Letter on Catholic Social Teaching and the U.S. Economy,* ##295-325.

18. *Economic Justice for All: Pastoral Letter on Catholic Social Teaching and the U.S. Economy,* ##178-182.

19. *Economic Justice for All: Pastoral Letter on Catholic Social Teaching and the U.S. Economy,* ##77-78.

20. *Economic Justice for All: Pastoral Letter on Catholic Social Teaching and the U.S. Economy,* ##75.

21. *Economic Justice for All: Pastoral Letter on Catholic Social Teaching and the U.S. Economy,* ##31-40.

Reflection Questions

1. The chapter opens with a challenge: How can we participate in shaping the new world that is emerging so that it will be more just, more revealing of the Reign of God among us?
   - What are the identifying marks of the Reign of God? Explain your answer.
   - What changes should be made in the world order to make it more reflective of God's presence, God's reign?
   - What changes should be made in healthcare services and institutions to accomplish this?
   - Do you perceive this moment in history as an especially graced time that allows room for radical conversion and societal healing that will focus our vision on the heart of the Christian life?

2. Economic pressures are forcing us to ask some fundamental questions. How do your respond to them?
   - What part does Catholic healthcare play in the larger healthcare picture?
   - How, honestly, is Catholic healthcare different?
   - What part does healthcare play in the nation's economy? What part should it play?
   - What part does the economy play in U.S. social and political life and culture? What part should it play?
   - In the future, will Catholic healthcare institutions minister primarily to the wealthy? What do you think can and should be done about this danger?

3. The chapter suggest that we can no longer leave justice issues to the social activists, that we are being forced to recognize that everyone is simultaneously engaged in justice issues at personal, interpersonal, and societal levels.
   - Are you conscious of the impact of your presence in your social setting? Explain.
   - In addition to the direct service you render, do you consider the social contexts of the human suffering, disease, and death you address?

- Have you
  - –Faced the reality of this time in healthcare?
  - –Grieved?
  - –Dealt with depression?
  - –Nurtured your identity?
  - –Accepted this moment in faith and with hope?
4. As we in healthcare cope with the identity crises of the Exilic period, we need a redemptive vision that will give us a lifegiving identity for the changed situation into which we are living.
   - What kind of relationships do you consider healthy and healing?
   - How can we model such relationships on the institutional, systematic, and societal level?

Epilogue

Immense problems are facing Catholic healthcare today. One healthcare worker has put it so clearly and forcefully that it deserves extended quotation:

Despite the advancement of modern medicine, millions of these...people are deprived of even the most basic form of healthcare. There is an unjust and uneven distribution of healthcare. The whole healthcare system is manipulated and held in the hands of the powerful—those who possess the power of wealth, social status, political influence and knowledge, control the planning and distribution of healthcare. Hence healthcare is primarily conditioned by the level of per capita income and socio-political power. The poor have no access to healthcare in the present economic and political system. Government policy on health services is unable to deal with health related problems of the poor in our society.

The health of the people cannot be seen in isolation. The problems of disease, malnutrition, high infant mortality, psychological oppression and the waste of human potential and resources are all linked with the socio-economic reality where poverty, exploitation by the moneylenders, low wages,...and control of the market by a few are again symptoms of an unjust social system of which the prevailing health system is but a part. Health for and by the people cannot become a reality fully except in a society that is "healthy" in its structures and its institutions. The question then is: how can community health work contribute to the transformation of the whole of society?[1]

This was written in India about India in 1982. It could be written about the United States of the late 1980s and into the 1990s. Solutions to the situation are anything but clear, and this book certainly cannot claim to provide them. Still, we can draw a few conclusions to serve as guidelines in our search for effective responses.

1. Healthcare and the problems facing it must be seen in their complex historical and societal context. Healthcare has had to learn through the centuries the importance and the nature of the interdependent physical systems that comprise the human body. Holistic medicine today is recalling our attention to the intricate role of the human spirit in bodily health and healing. It is equally important to realize that no person can be adequately diagnosed or understood without attention to the social groups, institutions, and societal conditions that shape his or her being. Personal health is societally conditioned and has societal impact. We overlook this fact only at the cost of failing in our full healing mission.

Healthcare personnel and delivery systems are also part of this social context. We are participants in the institutions and structure of society that generate the problems. We must keep a critical eye on the roles we play in the overall societal system and keep struggling to find ways to heal its diseased functioning.

2. The problems facing healthcare today are not only societal in their roots and ramifications, they are also deeply religious. Religion is not about a realm of life separate and distinct from our everyday "secular" involvements. It is not the specialized concern of pastoral care departments alone. It concerns a dimension of all of life; its fundamental meaning and value in relation to God and to our mission in life. As such, it involves us all.

The problem of healthcare for the poor has an added religious importance. Special love for and commitment to the poor is increasingly recognized to be at the heart of the Christian revelation. As the U.S. bishops' pastoral on the economy stated those who turn their backs on the poor turn their backs on God present and suffering in human history.[2]

3. Since the problems are religious in their root significance, our responses to them are profoundly religious actions. They put flesh and blood on our sense of religious mission. As

209

such, they should not be determined simply by the canons or codes of some school of management or marketing theory. Management and marketing principles must be incorporated into a much deeper, broader process of prayerful discernment in faith together.

4. We all must be involved in this process of discernment—laity and religious, administrators, all levels of healthcare workers, patients, representatives of society at large, and especially the poor. All bring important perspectives and background experience that should be heard and respected if God's action and invitation in the situation are to be interpreted faithfully. Such broad participation does not guarantee any sort of "pipeline to God," but it can embody the reverence for all God's children that Jesus modeled and called for. And it opens the possibility for a fuller grasp of God's revelation today, mediated as it is in the rich mosaic of human community interacting in history.

5. The discernment must include analysis of the structural societal forces shaping the problems before us. The skills of social, political, economic, and cultural analysis, therefore, can and must be developed insofar as possible by all participants so that justice can be done to the complexity of the situation.

6. This discernment process must give special attention to the experience and perspective of the poor. Attempts to solve the problems for the poor in a paternalistic manner do not do justice to the mission we are called to today. The analysis and responses developed must be shaped with the poor, and their assessments—so often ignored—should be given a privileged place.

7. To enter this process seriously and with integrity will affect every dimension of our lives and mission—from personal and institutional lifestyles to management, labor, and patient policy to political involvement. There is always great resistance to such changes. What is at stake here is our own liberation from our society's false values and the realization in our lives and institutions of the gospel values of solidarity with all, especially the poor.

8. Entering this process will involve us in the emerging mission of the church to U.S. society in response to the challenging revelation from God that it is discovering in the current socioeconomic situation. The peace pastoral and the pastoral on the economy sketch that revelation through themes of creation, covenant, and community set in the context of the purification

and conversion brought about by an experience of loss, of stripping, of exile. They call the U.S. church to this type of discerning effort to transform our society, to work for the peace and justice that are signs of true social health.

9. Finally, if our discerning responses to these problems are truly Catholic, they will link us more and more with our sisters and brothers around the world in mutually enriching relationships—especially with those in the Third World living often in desperate poverty and lacking the most basic healthcare.

How might such relationships be mutually enriching? In India one group of healthcare workers has developed an intriguing and successful program among the illiterate rural poor that requires few resources beyond what the people have available. The group goes to the poor communities, learns from them some of their health problems, and then invites them to send a representative for some basic healthcare training.

The training program for these village representatives focuses in the first two-week session on appropriate issues of basic hygiene and nutrition. The instructors may also provide some important tips on simple care for the most common diseases in the communities. After the session, the trainees return to share what they have learned with their communities. Since they are members of the communities, it is easier for them than for outsiders to win the people's trust. The goal of their training has not been to prepare them for incorporation into the healthcare system in what would inevitably be low level positions. Rather, it has been to prepare them to develop within their communities a variety of improved healthcare skills, drawing wherever possible on the folk medicine in the peoples' own culture and the natural medicinal plants and foods available where they live.

After a few months of experience, the new health workers return to the program to reflect on their experience, share their problems, learn more, and plan strategies for more effective community service. This time the educational component includes some guidance in how to analyze some of the social causes of their illness in the structures that shape and perpetuate their poverty.

Through several rounds of this work-reflection-education cycle, these health promoters have become effective leaders and community organizers. In summing up the program, Sara Kaithathara writes:

> Obviously institutions are always needed for health-care. But the concept has to be changed to a community approach which goes beyond sickness and health to family and community-related problems. This way, community health workers can be part of a system relevant to the people. Otherwise there remains a gap between the health workers, on the one side, and the health center and hospital on the other. This can be bridged by the continuing education of all involved together with decentralization of functions and responsibilities. This has been our experience.[3]

Perhaps an approach similar to this one could and should become important in our responses to the current situation in the United States. The struggles for legislative change being undertaken by healthcare institutions and systems must go on. Still, we must remember that they go on in the halls of power and are usually bounded by the limited horizons and aspirations of the wealthy and powerful. Significant and lasting solutions will only be found when the poor's experience, voices, skills, and power are unleashed and we work with them to heal our society.

Perhaps this epilogue and one of the key underlying messages of this book can be summed up in a few words. It is important for us to remember that the poor are not just healthcare's problem. They are also its privilege. To paraphrase the words of an administrator friend of mine recently, we are only beginning to realize that we need the poor and the Third World even more than they need us.

The poor are far, far more than a vexing problem or even a threat to Catholic healthcare today. At a deeper level they are the embodiment of Christ reaching out to us in invitation. They hold the key to the future of our Christian integrity and mission.

Footnotes
  1. Volken, Henry, Ajo, Kumar, and Sara Kaithathara, *Learning From the Rural Poor: Shared Experiences of the Mobile Orientation Training Team,* Indian Social Institute, New Delhi, 1982, p. 64.
  2. *Economic Justice for All: Pastoral Letter on Catholic Social Teaching and the U.S. Economy,* National Conference of Catholic Bishops, U.S. Catholic Conference, Washington, DC, 1986, #44.
  3. *Learning From the Rural Poor: Shared Experiences of the Mobile Orientation Training Team,* p. 89.

Index

About the Authors

James E. Hug, SJ, is the executive director of the Center of Concern, Washington, DC, and its former director of research. Hug spent four and one-half years at the Woodstock Theological Center also in Washington. He focuses on research and education on the issues of faith and economic justice, Catholic social teaching, the future of the healthcare ministry, and theological reflection in the work of justice. Hug has a PhD in Christian ethics from the University of Chicago and is a frequent author and speaker on healthcare and social and economic justice.

Peter J. Henriot, SJ, is working in grass roots development projects in the Diocese of Monze in Zambia. He was formerly director of the Center of Concern. He taught at the Joint Center for Urban Studies of MIT-Harvard and at Seattle University. Henriot engages in research and educational efforts on questions of political economy and social value issues in a global society; participates in programs devoted to promoting church response to justice issues; and analyzes U.S. policies toward the developing world, peace issues, and social programs. He has a PhD in political science from the University of Chicago and has a long list of publications.

Joseph Holland is executive director of PILLAR, the Pallotine Institute for Lay Leadership and Apostolic Research and has spent many years involved in the promotion of lay leadership in the Church. Holland was a long time staff member of the Center of Concern. He is also writing and lecturing on spirituality and post-modern culture.